AF510862

Building Digital Health Competencies in Developing Countries

BUILDING DIGITAL HEALTH COMPETENCIES IN DEVELOPING COUNTRIES

Sara D. Garduño-Diaz and Friedrich Huth

Delve
PUBLISHING

www.delvepublishing.com

Building Digital Health Competencies in Developing Countries

Sara D. Garduño-Diaz and Friedrich Huth

Delve Publishing

224 Shoreacres Road

Burlington, ON L7L 2H2

Canada

www.delvepublishing.com

Email: orders@arclereducation.com

ISBN: 978-1-77469-536-4 (Hardcover)

ABOUT THE AUTHORS

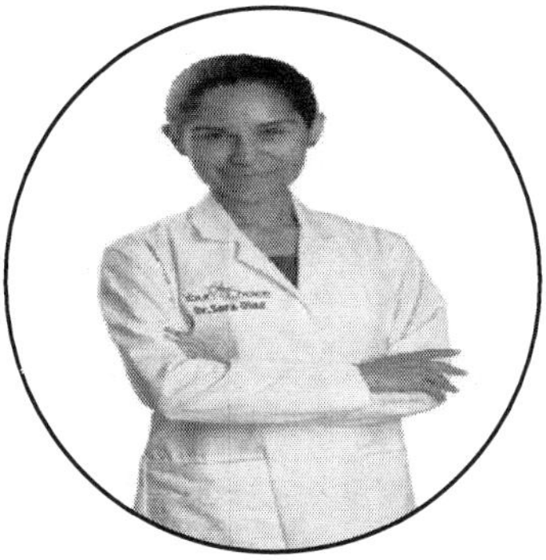

Sara D. Garduño-Diaz has a background in nutrition with a PhD in Nutrition and Food Science from the University of Leeds, United Kingdom; she has further specialized in Sports Nutrition with the International Olympics Committee, Switzerland. Dr Garduño-Diaz has worked as Research Fellow for several EU-funded research projects and was awarded research grants from CONACYT (Mexico) and the BBSRC (UK). She currently consults for various startups in Europe and the US in the areas of Nutrition and Product Development.

Dr Garduño-Diaz sits on the editorial board of various international journals, including the Journal of Obesity and Weight Management, E Cronicon Nutrition, Research in Health Science, and Insights in Nutrition and Dietetics. She is the author of over 50 peer-reviewed publications and 10 books. Her research interests include the dietary patterns of migrant populations and their impact on health, as well as investigating the environmental factors that influence food selection.

Dr. Garduño-Diaz is a member of the Academy of Nutrition and Dietetics, the American Overseas Dietetics Association, Professionals in Nutrition for Exercise & Sport, and the World Public Health Nutrition Association, for whom she is a member of the executive committee.

With over 15 years of experience in the field of nutrition, and having lived and worked in various continents, Dr Garduño-Diaz's approach to food is one of integrating strategies to design individual programs based on her client's wellness needs. Dr Garduño-Diaz advocates for real food and the art of eating.

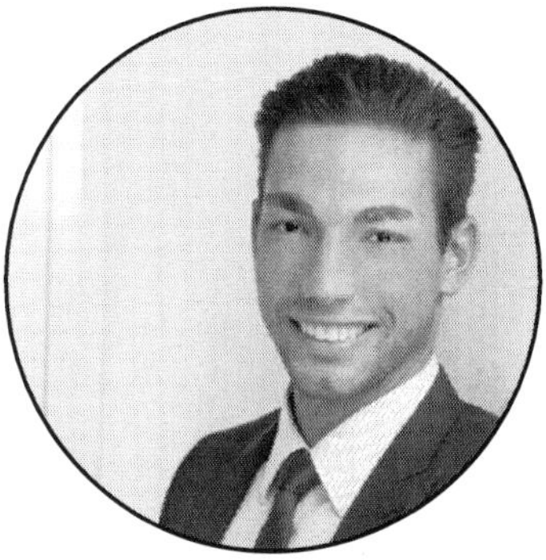

Friedrich Huth has a background in Business Economics with a Master's Degree in Business Administration from the University of Brandenburg, Germany. He further specialized in Corporate Finance at the Institute of International Studies at the Ramkhamhaeng University in Bangkok. When an arthrosis diagnosis ended his career as a professional Athlete and Captain of the German Youth Basketball National Team at an early age, he dedicated his life to helping a variety of small and medium sized companies grow their business as Operations, Marketing and Finance Manager while personally exploring measures to cure his joint-condition and regain his physical abilities. Thus, he started working on functional nutrition in 2017 when he became a first line member of Her1, an Ecommerce startup for Nutritional Supplements. Currently he is responsible for a unit of consultants with focus on German Companies in the Agriculture, Life Science, Pharmaceutical & Chemical Industries. Due to his professional environment he is exposed to first line insights on the practices and strategies of the main players in related fields to modern food production.His approach to digital health is based on his personal nutrition-induced full recovery from a condition that was prognosed to be irreversible, mixed with over 6 years of professional experience in economic fields.

TABLE OF CONTENTS

LIST OF FIGURES

LIST OF TABLES

LIST OF BOXES

SUMMARY

It has been proposed by the World Health Organization that three intrinsic components are required for a health system to perform at an optimal level (WHO, 2000):

1. The system must improve the health of the population,
2. There must be fair financial contribution,
3. Responsiveness must be timely

In combination, these three areas of optimization may derive hefty benefits from the implementation of their corresponding digital components, both in the developing and developed world. Nevertheless, before the setup of functional digital tools is the compulsory development of competency. In this case, digital health competency.

In the context of this book, digital health competency refers to "the use of information and communications technology in support of health and health-related fields" (WHO, 2019). The concept of digital health may appear overwhelming upon first glance. Numerous health care services as well as providers employ classic paper-based systems for information, and taking up technology is not within the possibilities and expertise of several health systems. Initiating with digital health, nevertheless, is similar to implementing any novel program, often with more questions than answers. To begin, especially for practitioners with limited or no background with technology, comes "What can digital health really do?"

The correct answers may not always be technology, yet if it is, an abundance of informed decisions must be taken. Various of these decisions center around trade-offs, and even though no "right" answer really exists, some options have greater context-relevance and are more feasible than others when considering developing countries. Taking up a participatory angle to developing the envisioned digital tool with end users is paramount. Empowering health care professionals to try out a concept or model a situation with the potential digital health tool to potentially outphase their current systems can shine light on key insights. It is then possible to fine tune top ideas into even better answers with the added perspective of those who will be affected.

Regardless of the potential of digital health to provide possibilities to improve the quality, efficiency and safety of healthcare, takeup of digital tools and technologies has not been a quick process, in part due to lacking digital health literacy.

For health systems to make full usage of digital tools, a capable, digitally savvy workforce is required. Various existing digital health products have already been proven worthy, are already available, and are being tailored to country-specific requirements. Nevertheless, a global framework that rallies resources, experts, and strategies to carry out the true potential of digital health is only at a nascent stage.

CHAPTER 1

DEFINING DIGITAL HEALTH COMPETENCIES

CONTENTS

INTRODUCTION

Regardless of digital health giving way to numerous opportunities to increase the quality, efficiency and safety of healthcare across all disciplines, the implementation of digital tools and technologies has been slow in the take up, in part as a result of lacking digital health literacy. So that healthcare systems may optimally use said technologies, a competent, digitally literate population is needed. Digital health has already created opportunities for the future modification of health services, doing so by empowering people to manage their health with increasing effectiveness, allowing for more accurate diagnosis, and measuring the impact of policies, among various benefits (WHO, 2018).

Health education, including digital health competency, that is accessible, structured and comprehensive is warranted. What remains to be fully grasped however, is which digital health competencies are needed for health professionals to implement and make use of digital health in initial and continuous care. This understanding depends on a variety of factors such as the type of technologies used, the care delivery personnel involved, and the degree to which the environment has developed digitally thus far.

It can be said that digital health (DH) began with the progressive conversion of patients' information from physical to electronic files (Coiera, 2011), until keeping medical history in digital form became the common form of nonverbal communication in the health sector (O'Leary et al., 2011). The detailed allowance and quickness of digital record keeping allowed for the possibility to retain and systematically analyze a significant amount of clinical information, making way to two innovative fields: the analysis of big data, fostered by distributed learning (Deist et al., 2020), and the -omics boom, ranging from genomics (Obermeyer and Lee, 2017) to radiomics (Gatta et al., 2029). From this point on, a monodisciplinary information and communications technology approach is insufficient across all areas of health care (Tagliaferri et al., 2016; Tagliaferri et al., 2028; Meldolesi et al., 2014). Moreover, as it is the case of companies from other fields outside of medicine and paramedical support, the digitalisation of healthcare professionals and institutions must be guided by dedicated and competent individuals including emerging required roles to be covered such as digital officers and remote clinical carers. However, taking into consideration the complexity of health care dynamics and the need for clinical decision-making pathways, a medical background remains a required baseline in need of additional digital competency development (Burki,

2019). In tandem, those on the receiving end of health care services must also become competent in the digitalization of the field. From appointment booking, to wearable technologies for biomarkers, technology is now an intrinsic part of health care and maintenance.

Box 1. What is Digital Health?

Digital health refers to the application of information and communications technologies, computer science, and data in a systematic manner to allow for informed decision-making by the public, healthcare professionals, and health institutions, so as to improve resilience to adverse health conditions and achieve health and wellness for everyone. The Classification of Digital-Health Interventions published by the World Health Organization (WHO) lists more than 80 digital technology applications for reinforcing health institutions as well as systems, and categorizes them in accordance to their main target population, which covers these:

- Technologies oriented towards the client, including those that prompt timely reminders for appointment and health management, communicate alerts for upcoming health-related events, and/or allow for payments;
- Technologies oriented towards the provider, including those that allow for the identification and tabulation of users; keeping of health history files; discussion and decision-making for care professionals; orientation towards additional or different services; planning and appointment keeping; further education; and the handling of biological indicator values and results, diagnostics, and imaging, and "virtual health," covering monitoring remotely and digital medicine;
- Technologies oriented towards managers, covering those that provide support to the management of people operations, supply-chains, communication of public health-related activities, civil registries and key statistics, funds from the public and private sector, as well as facilities;
- Technologies oriented as data services, including those that allow the listing, management, analytics, coding, exchange, interoperability, and application of information; and location-tracking.

As communicated in the draft WHO 2020–2024 Global Strategy on Digital Health, the concept of "digital health" makes reference to "the field of knowledge and practice associated with any aspect of adopting digital technologies to improve health," and covers the subdomains of eHealth, medical informatics, health informatics, telemedicine, digital health and mHealth, in addition to data-analytics, big data, and artificial intelligence. In this context, the following terms are defined as:

eHealth: The cost-effective and secure use of information and communications technologies in support of health and health-related fields, including health care services, health surveillance, health literature, and health education, knowledge and research.

infodemic: An infodemic is an acute outpouring of information, including potentially misleading or inaccurate information that, in a digital, hyper- connected society such as the present one, is likely bound to accompany every epidemic or acute health crisis.

telemedicine: The delivery of health care services, where distance is a critical factor, by all healthcare professionals using information and communications technologies for the exchange of valid information for diagnosis, treatment and prevention of disease and injuries, research and evaluation, and the continuing education of health care workers, with the aim of advancing the health of individuals and communities.

digital health: The field of knowledge and practice associated with the development and use of digital technologies to improve health. Digital health expands the concept of eHealth to include digital consumers, with a wider range of smart-devices and connected equipment. It also encompasses other uses of digital technologies for health such as the Internet of things, artificial intelligence, big data and robotics.

digital divide: Refers to the gap between demographics and regions that have access to modern information and communications technology and those that do not or have restricted access. This technology can include the telephone, television, personal computers and the Internet.

digital hospital: The digital hospital provides services within and outside the hospital walls shifting away from the facility-based delivery of care to a smart virtual network of care centered on the patient, embedded in the health continuum.

health data: The systematic application of information and communications technologies, computer science, and data to support informed decision- making by individuals, the health workforce, and health systems, to strengthen resilience to disease and improve health and wellness. It includes all data pertaining to the health status of a data subject which reveal information relating to the past, current or future physical or mental health status of the data subject. This includes information about the natural person collected in the course of the registration for, or the provision of, health care services to that natural person; a number, symbol or particular assigned to a natural person to uniquely identify the natural person for health purposes.

*h*ealth information system: A system that integrates data collection, processing, reporting, and use of the information necessary for improving health service effectiveness and efficiency through better management at all levels of health services.

Another area of DH is artificial intelligence (AI) (Allen et al., 2019). Covering a range including pattern recognition (Topol, 2019) and all the way to process identification and enhancing (Gatta et al., 2018), AI is highly grasping for many scientists and high-tech businesses. Nevertheless, a significant challenge of AI is the operators' constant lack of understanding of the steps that lead to the outcomes: is it possible to trust an algorithm to "decide" which management plan for a health condition will be followed without a full grasp of it? AI is, hence, a paramount topic in the area of ethics as well. This has been documented in the "Rome call for AI Ethics", a declaration supported by some of the largest companies worldwide and the Pontifical Academy for Life, where a new name has been proposed to address the application of ethics within an algorithm: the "algor-ethics" (Rome call for ethics, 2020).

Additionally, DH is not just made up of various high-tech tools for models of predictions, but permits tailored clinical selection and optimization of the clinical human intelligence component. Numerous applications are created daily for communication and remote consultation and niche businesses are developed to deliver online services for remote medical evaluation of the care receivers (Bhavnani et al., 2016; Fionda et al., 2019).

Moreover, with the COVID-19 pandemic, people are becoming aware of the limitations of their corresponding health care systems (Keesara et al., 2020). With this in mind, DH's capacity to provide tools, instruments and services is noteworthy: from the application of AI(Allam and Jones, 2020) to the possibility of proposing remote consultation to replace the traditional clinical examination so as to contain possible risks of infection or contagion (Geenhalgh et al., 2020). The relevance of DH is fastly increasing. Hence, governments and businesses are highly recommended to invest strongly in it and direct political decision making in its favor (Collins and Varmus, 2015). Additionally, increasing literature demonstrates the impact of high-tech applications in medicine (Obermeyer and Emanuel, 2016). For that reason, a digital-competent profile is recommended for any professional involved in the various fields of health (Fridsma, 2018; Mai et al., 2018; Han et al., 2019; Mandl and Kohane, 2008; Han et al., 2005; Benwell et al., 2017). Regardless of its exponential development in complexity, to date a specific training course in DH is not required in the majority of MD graduation programs (Jidkov et al., 2019; Lennon et al., 2017; Marotta, 2017).

There can be disruptions in a health system when digital transformation occur; nevertheless, technologies including the use of internet, cyber care, monitoring remotely, AI, analysis of big data, blockchain, wearables, virtual platforms, tools allowing data exchange and safekeeping, and tools enabling information collection from afar, as well the swapping of data and disseminating of timely information across health systems, creating ongoing care have demonstrated potential to improve health outcomes by enhancing diagnosis, facilitating decision taking for treatment based on data, the implementation of digital therapeutics, clinical trials, self-management of care and care centered around individuals, as well as creating more evidence-based information, skills and competence for professionals to support health care.

Digital health competency development should be a required part of health prioritization and benefit individuals and communities in a way that is ethical, safe, secure, reliable, equitable and sustainable. Such development must be set forward with principles of transparency, accessibility, scalability, replicability, interoperability, privacy, security and confidentiality.

The adaptation of technology and digital competency to the domestic health system is causing some struggles to policymakers, while international advocacy groups are only just beginning to establish the principles, practices, and tools to help late uptakers and developing nations in keeping up. For a successful international digital health framework to be implemented, it is necessary for low- and middle-income countries to enter into global partnerships on key foundations, including:

- national strategies
- skill development
- establishing infrastructure
- developing governance that balances innovation and data protection

4A world-wide digital health framework is only at an initial stage. As can be understood, policymakers across nations are initially dealing with the hefty hurdle of tailoring technology to their particular domestic health frameworks. And global bodies are only now initiating the development of common principles, best practices, and tools to assist late adaptors and countries under development to strive to match those countries leading the way. COVID-19 has highlighted the importance of global cooperation and collaboration to ensure the interconnected health of all.

Low and middle-income country (LMIC) policymakers and their international health and development stakeholders must zoom in on foundational issues—including a national digital health strategy, digital competency development, information and communications technology (ICT) infrastructure, and data governance—so as to put in place effective domestic and international digital health frameworks. This book aims to support all stakeholders involved in doing this.

Digital health frameworks must be regularly updated with novel digital health technologies, be applicable to low- and middle-income countries as well as those more developed nations, and include overlooked health care worker groups in addition to those at the receiving end of healthcare.

Box 2. Key Messages.

The adoption of digital solutions offers unique opportunities to optimize health systems and address the challenges of timely responsiveness to health requirements. This includes existing chronic conditions and sudden occurrences such as epidemics of infectious diseases.

Even so, the various fields of health and medicine fall behind other institutions in grasping the potential of digital technologies. Regardless of significant efforts and some promising national thiumphs, health systems in most of the EU and OECD countries remain yet to experience a strong digital transformation. Consider the following:

- Various existing datasets and health services remain to be electronically connected, impeding the flow of vital information – a serious problem, for example, during sudden pandemics.
- The implementation of digital health and remote solutions is not wide-ranging, often maintained only for exceptional cases, independent of amounting evidence of beneficial outcomes, slowing down progress in providing care to hard-to-reach patients, facilitating access, and pivoting from reactive approaches to maintaining health.
- The implementation of analytical tools using diverse data and technologies including AI is just emerging at a slow pace, regardless of the complexity of medical procedures and the resulting high dependence on stepwise information to address challenges.

The obstacles to the uptake of digitalization in health are not just technical, but additionally institutional and organizational. While stakeholders and policy makers must commit to ongoing investment in interoperability and the setup of an adaptable digital architecture, they must additionally guarantee prompt modernisation of policy and governance frameworks. The most pressing which are:

- securing effective approaches and policies across sectors;
- prompt adjustment of legislative and financial frameworks for the digital era;
- providing suitable support for health workerS.

Digital health building blocks

Independently from the possible upsides of digital health, a limited number of nations have set off needed policies, programs, or strategies for a full utilization of said benefits. The 2019 Global Digital Health Index analyzes the degree of readiness and uptake of digital health in 22 countries at various stages of economic development (GDHI, 2020). Additionally, the Index measures the preparedness of the greater health system to be able to take on and roll out digital health interventions. The Index is developed in accordance to components of the WHO and International Telecommunications Union (ITU) eHealth Strategy Framework, which employs 19 indicators in 7 policy categories:

- leadership and governance;
- strategy and investment;
- services and applications;
- standards and interoperability;
- infrastructure;
- legislation, policy and compliance; and
- workforce.

The Index highlights that while numerous nations have national digital health strategies, the majority are missing national digital health architectures, health information exchanges, as well as data standards, all of which limit the potential advantages of digital technologies.

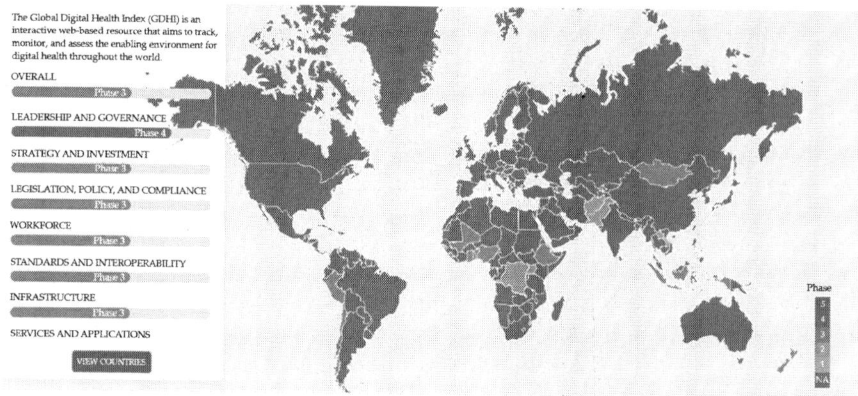

Figure 1. State of Digital Health Around the World.

Source: index.digitalhealthidex.org, 2022

International information sharing between nations' frameworks for data management—in so permitting data flow, and corresponding digital products, to move across jurisdictions—is paramount in optimizing the advantages of digital health. This information exchange allows institutions to combine larger, more valuable datasets for investigation, and leverage cloud services to provide health care between borders. For businesses involved in coming up with and providing digital health products and services, international interoperability is vital for their survival, as it builds economies of scale. For stakeholders and individuals, this translates into stronger care-sector competition, and a hand into a wider range of healthcare services. This is why policymakers must consider needs regionally and globally when contemplating domestic digital health and data governance policies.

When discussing a digital health setup, interoperability is the term used for technical and legal factors that hinder the different involved bodies in the collection, sharing, and analyzing of data since they normally exist in non-standardized form and are kept over isolated databases with software that is incompatible from one to the other. This is a connected, albeit additional, component of global interoperability within digital health. The goal of improved domestic interoperability is to assure effortless communication across different IT systems via compatible data standards, in accordance with international interoperability, and to guarantee data transfers between different countries.

The localization of data must be avoided as entities utilize information to create value—and the majority can only optimize that value when information can flow freely independent of borders. The transfer of information is paramount to the utilization of AI and big data for novell health and medical research, the creation and application of real-world data from individual devices including smart watches, international virus and disease surveillance, the distance delivery of health services to smart devices via apps, and doctor-patient interactions. Numerous firms and entities that conduct operations across multiple regions demonstrate how cross-border information exchange is key to their work.

As digital health competency is a prolongation of health literacy, it is affected by similar limits and contradictions, and the international scenario of access to modern health information is incomplete.

On one side, people (including medical doctors) are already quite involved in searching for information and answers in the health space, and globally there is a significant amount of health-related information traffic.

According to recent WHO data, 80% of health-related queries are carried out on Google or other search engines, and one out of 20 searches on Google is connected to health. In the United States, 72% of adults with internet access search for information about their health (in comparison to 60% in Europe).

Internet users, nevertheless, are often drowned in an information overload. More recent Google searches throw back over two billion results for "cancer" and almost 600 million for "diabetes" (note that these results were, respectively, 575 million and 250 million in 2017).

On the other hand, the WHO reported that 53% of the world's population is not on line (0-25% in the US and most of Europe, 26-50% in some European countries). Hence, there is the risk that the people most at risk are overlooked during the transition and that existing health inequalities experienced by populations who have lower levels of digital health literacy can be worsened.

Digital health literacy today

Considering the context given thus far, how is digital health competency being developed today, and who are the drivers in the field?

Worldwide, WHO is augmenting its focus on building digital health competency, nowadays referring to "the ability to seek, find, understand, and appraise health information from electronic sources and apply the knowledge gained to addressing or solving a health problem".

In accordance with this definition, digital health competency seems to exclusively refer to the use of digital tools to access overall health information. It does not include the key aspect of becoming literate about digital health.

As part of its original definition, WHO covered digital health literacy among the components of the Digital Health Ecosystem, as well as digital health, telemedicine, big data and governance interventions. Over the past few years, it has made available timely documents, including *Digital Technologies: Shaping the Future of Primary Health Care* (2018) and the first *WHO Guideline Recommendations on Digital Interventions for Health System Strengthening (*2019).

During the past twenty years, the countries belonging to the EU and OECD have created a significant movement towards developing and making better electronic files and databases within their healthcare systems. Currently, part of essential national (or regional) health databases, including hospital visitors data, information on emergency care, primary care information, formal long term health information, or prescription drugs information are within reach and employed in the daily management of care service provision in most countries. During the past five years, as an example, the availability and quality of the national primary care information records have notoriously improved due to the wider uptake of electronic health records among general medicine doctors, despite some countries continuing to stay behind (European Commission, 2018).

Nevertheless, the information records of various segments of healthcare systems in a nation remain to be communicated across systems electronically. Effectively, it ends up being the patients – or their family members – who transmit information about their management and condition history across the healthcare system, and health care practitioners remain in wait for a more effective setup where the correct information is available at the required time (OECD, 2019).

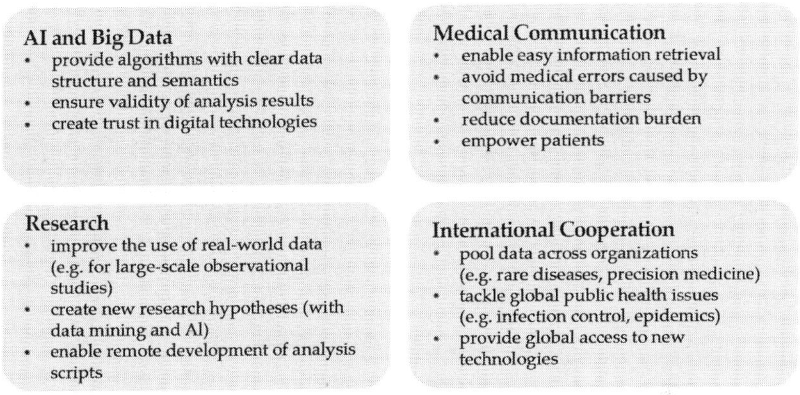

Figure 2. How interoperability improves digital medicine.

Source: Lehne et al., 2019

COMPONENTS OF DIGITAL HEALTH

While no single definition exists for digital health, it is generally agreed that the term makes reference to an all encompassing term covering eHealth, in turn generally defined as "the use of information and communications technology in support of health and health-related fields", in addition to up and coming fields of advance computer sciences in the areas of "big data", -omics and AI (WHO, 2019).

An analysis of the current status of global health systems has reported diversity between countries, with lower income countries being left behind (Rice et al., 2012). Existing, albeing limited, data from low and middle income countries reports that digital health competencies in the provision of medical attention is likely to be ignored and many times lacks meeting people's non-medical demands (Groenevegen et al., 2005). Nowadays, increased interest in assessing patient's experience with medical care services in low and middle-income countries is peaking, with the objective of determining the degree of satisfaction of healthcare system users (Valentine et al., 2003; Rice et al., 2012; Tippawan et al., 2012; Tolib et al., 2017).

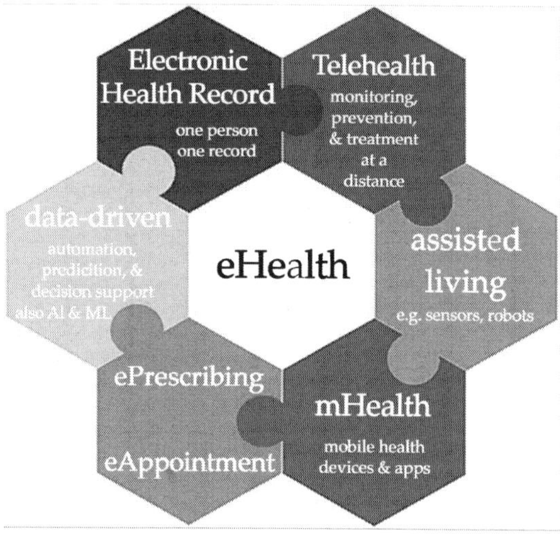

Figure 3. Defining Digital Health.

Source: eHealth Ireland, 2022

Health care digitization is quickly undergoing an evolutionary process, with ciber information and remote applications for digital devices having a key role in the delivery of medical care. In tandem with said modifications, the competency to search, select, evaluate, and apply medical information found on-line as well as digital applications related to health management have become essential for the public. Said combined set of skills are referred to as digital has been shown in various studies, demonstrating that individual's self-perceived skill set when it comes to the utilization of information available on-line has an impact on their health and their quality of care, and when such skills are found lacking, the outcomes may be adverse (Hsu et al., 2014; Neter et al., 2012). Hsu et al. (2014) reported that digital health competency is linked to numerous forms of health behavior, amongst which are listed healthy eating, exercise, and sleep behavior. Neter and Brainin (2012) showed connections between digital health competency and the likelihood of presenting chronic diseases, perceived self-management skills, and better self-perceived understanding of health conditions, symptomatology, and management options.

A relevant instrument for the measurement of digital health competency is key for the examination of the impact of these skills, both on a personal level and at a community level. At a personal level—as an example, in routine clinical practice—a measurement instrument could provide backup decisions regarding the extent to which a person is able to utilize a specific digital health tool with the corresponding interventions (Chang et al., 2004; Chan et al., 2011). In addition, it can generate feedback to guide and educate users who require support in utilizing internet-based health tools (Xie, 2011; Car et al., 2011). At a community level, a suitable measurement tool can give insight regarding at-risk subgroups that present additional challenges in implementing health care, because of its digitization. As an example, existing studies have reported that digital health competency is linked to socio demographics including age, education, and income (Neter et al., 2012; Chung et al., 2015; Chesser et al., 2016), while research has also shown that some communities do not have the competency to employ internet-based health instruments for their own gain and might thus become underserved (Chang et al., 2004; Chesser et al., 2016). More detailed information into populations at risk of low digital health competency can make way to the development and tailoring of health technologies for these specific groups (Change et al., 2004; Botte et al. 2008).

Considering a global setting, digital health is defined as "the field of knowledge and practice associated with the development and use of digital to improve health". This consideration includes eHealth, in accordance with the definition found in the report by the Director-General of the WHO (WHO, 2020). Digital health builds on the concept of eHealth to encompass digital users, with a greater coverage of smart and connected devices. It includes other uses of digital technologies for medical care and wellness as well, including the extensive and continuous use of the internet, advanced computing, analysis of Big Data, AI including machine learning, as well as robotics.

In turn, the FDA defines digital health as "mobile health (mHealth), health information technology (IT), wearable devices, digital health and telemedicine, and personalized medicine." The technologies used in digital health cover digital therapeutics, mobile apps, AI, machine learning software, and sensors, among various more.

Nevertheless, digital health competency must be user-focused in order to support the user's health in an impactful manner. As a way to illustrate this concept, when a user asks for a specific drug that lacks sufficient efficacy evidence, facilitating the prescription is not always user-centered care.

4Digital health innovations can be most effective when it strengthens user-carer connections, allows for useful communication that can be acted upon, educates users regarding self-management of health conditions, encourages user engagement, or manages additional positive results.

Digital health competency benefits may include:

- Reduced human error and increased efficiency
- Reduction in stigmas
- Increased patient satisfaction
- Improved access to care
- Minimized friction in communications
- Increased engagement of users
- Lower costs
- Greater speed of services
- Reduced needs and burdens of staffing
- More effective billing experience
- Greater consistency
- Smoother workflows
- Allowance for personalization
- Greater quality of care

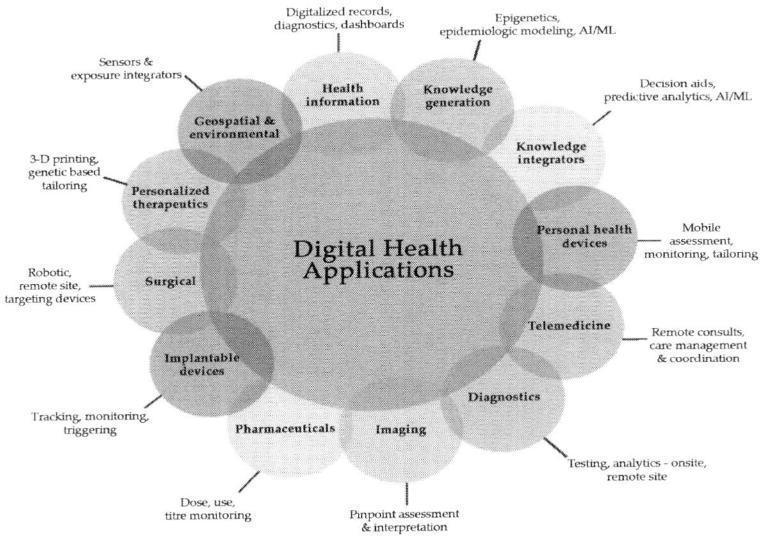

Figure 4. Applications of Digital Technology on Health and Health Care.

Source: National Academy of Medicine. 2019. Digital Health Action Collaborative, NAM Leadership Consortium: Collaboration for a Value & Science-Driven Health System.

Reducing the digital health competency gap for health results is a key obstacle made harder by frequently evolving technology. Towards the end of 2018, the Digital Frontiers Institute put together a seminar series called "Digital Health: Building a Future Proof Workforce" to explore said topic, covering the competencies required and identifying existing gaps (Mechael and Edelman, 2019). A couple of the key gaps highlighted were:

- lack of digital health leaders, managers, and policymakers;
- missing digital health program designers and implementers;
- required architects, programmers, engineers, and data scientists;
- development of digital health skills for health professionals including doctors, nurses, and administrators.

These points identify the problem areas to be covered in order to secure sufficient staff with the suitable technical expertise for back-end IT system design and operations. As an example, for sustainable infrastructure of digital health, participants at the Digital Frontiers Institute highlighted the skills needed to roll out and upkeep hardware, software, and connectivity, in addition to the ability to build basic, reusable infrastructure that allows for economies of scale.

Targeted skills that aid health systems to have greater adaptability to evolving technology cover data scientists; visualization analysts; enterprise architects; data architects and modelers; machine learning and natural language processing specialists; systems networking and communications experts, including human to machine interaction; and security and cryptography experts.

The World Health Organization's Action Plan for the Global Strategy of Digital Health 2020–2024 suggests for all WHO member states to commit to increasing training capacity, encompassing the capacity of tertiary institutions and developing relevant training programs. In turn, th 2019 Global Digital Health Index identifies momentum towards the development of digital health, health informatics, health information systems, and biomedical informatics degree programs; these begin showing promising outputs in the development of specialized digital health workers, particularly in nations including Bangladesh, Chile, Ethiopia, Kuwait, Malaysia, Peru, Portugal, Sri Lanka, Thailand, and Uganda. Individual descriptions of the status of the development of digital health competency in these countries can be found throughout the rest of this book. Nevertheless, the majority of countries have reported insufficient training to cover the existing demand, and digital considerations remain to be properly reflected in the career programs of civil workers across all health fields.

Governments, donors, and other stakeholders are urged to develop unified templates for the identification and response to the most-pressing skills required, and to match them with a corresponding list of best practices and training programs for the development of competencies in workers. These may take the form of a "lowest common skill set" in order for low and middle income countries (LMIC) to be able to begin working on addressing the most critical digital competency gaps. There are likely to be various common factors across LMICs, translating into a possible common template that could be useful in avoiding wasting both time and financial investments from otherwise having each country creating its own tools for digital health competency development. As part of this template response, regional and multilateral health expert bodies as well as relevant donors and private-sector stakeholders are urged to collaborate with local governments in identifying and prioritizing the most-pressing areas that act as bottlenecks to improved outcomes.

Box 3. Digital Health Development in Bangladesh

Bangladesh has achieved noteworthy development in digital health over the past few years. Making use of one of the biggest deployments of the open-source District Health Information Software 2 (DHIS2) worldwide, Bangladesh currently possesses a national health data warehouse for the public sector. Data from what used to be incomplete information systems is currently compiled in a collective information repository, allowing for information exchange for medical information systems and optimal making of decisions. Continuous work is being carried out to develop lifetime digital medical records for all citizens that are able to be shared across medical care facilities. Lengthy tailoring of open-source software has created the groundwork for a national digital networking system.

Initiatives have targeted the development of electronic solutions to help priorities including reinforcing the medical care system as an entirety in addition to supporting precise technical interventions, such as making the civil registration and vital statistics system better than its previous versions. Electronic solutions have also backed up the country's health care professionals' strategy by way of a compilation of registries that digitally captures and keeps human resource data for the entire medical sector, covering monitoring the attendance of employees by way of low-cost biometric fingerprint time-attendance machines. Users are prompted to engage in modeling health services through an on-line complaints and suggestions system. In addition, a novel system to increase health awareness through public digital displays has begun in Dhaka. Hefty support at the top political level has been key to the success of initiatives to implement said innovations.

The endeavor has also created strong and enthusiastic proponents of digital health competency development, targeting further development and expansion of the current systems. It also helps harness the vast quantities of data amassed at the central information repository via big data analysis, AI and machine learning (WHO, 2019).

Table 1. Principles for Digital Development

1. Design with the user in mind
2. Understanding the current context
3. Design for scale
4. Sustainability in development
5. Develop based on data
6. Use Open Standards, Open Data, Open Source, and Open Innovation
7. Reuse and improve
8. Consider privacy and security
9. Be collaborative

Credit: Principles of Digital Development

The term "competence" is multifactorial and in some cases vague, including knowledge, skills, performance, attitudes and values (Cowan et al., 2005; Mikkonen et al., 2018). In addition, a framework of professional competence has been proposed in the past by Cheetham and Chivers (1998) and covers five areas of competences as follows:

- cognitive (including informal tacit knowledge, knowledge and understanding);
- functional (including skills and know-how);
- personal (behavioral competencies);
- ethical (including appropriate personal and professional values); and
- meta-competences (including learning, reflection and the ability to cope with uncertainty).

The definition of digital competence may be considered as "the confident, critical, collaborative and creative use of information technology" (European Commission, 2016). Digital competence is covered by the basic information and communication technology (ICT) skillset, which allows a person to access, retrieve, produce and present information—in addition to being able to communicate in collaborative networks—through the use of the internet (Vuorikari et al., 2016).

Box 4. Digital Health Development in Chile

The increasing cost of medical care in Chile and Latin America has created the demand for a more efficient and cost-effective healthcare system. Appointments, referrals, missed appointments, misdiagnoses, and ambulance calls create an expensive burden on the system in addition to costing a significant quantity of time and money. Medical care that is value-based has the objective to make cost- effective, science-based medical care accessible, in addition to addressing patient values that improve life expectancy and lead to a higher life quality. This path could help track people remotely, reduce the risk of disease, and give accurate drug and alternative management options to existing health conditions.

The developing Chilean approach to developing digital health competency amongst its national population benefits not only the recipients of care but also health providers, and related stakeholders within the wider care system. Remote access to physicians is one of the most impactful answers to the unsustainable demand on the Chilean healthcare system in existence today. It could further aid with the implementation of more tailored patient care by providing physicians with the time to allow for longer appointments via telephone and video consultations with users. In turn, this could lower waiting times in public hospitals and private clinics (Barra Nova, 2021).

Digital health competency has been defined in the past as comprising suitable skills in implementing digital technology to supply high-quality ethical care to the user, social and communication skills to utilize digital technology in the prevention of adverse health effects, diagnostics and multi-option management, willingness and motivation to make use of digital technology in a professional setting, and collegial and organizational backup for the enhancement of positive experiences in digitalization (Konttila et al., 2018). Existing reports of users of digital health services have reported both negative and positive feedback, with the negative points most often linked to the perception of a lack of competence in communicating with users through portals (Laukka et al., 2020), management and screening algorithms threatening their medical competency (Odendaal et al. 2020) and questions over whether digital health improves medical care for the users (Ross et al., 2016). Challenges such as lacking design of services and careless adoption of process in addition to a lack of access to digital tools have been highlighted as slowing down the use of digital technology in medical care as well as existing concerns over technology removing time from direct patient attention and leading to extra stress originating from malfunctioning systems (Brown et al., 2020).

Contrary to these points, the positive highlights of digital health have been linked to digital competency and the trust that digital health carries strong benefits for its users (Odendaal et al. 2020, Ross et al., 2016). In addition, the acceptance and implementation of digital health are impacted by competence, abilities and experience (Ross et al., 2016). Thus, healthcare companies must ascertain that health care providers are competent in digital health as a response to constantly changing roles and responsibilities, along with the increasing importance of digital technology in medical care (Nazeha et al., 2020; While & Dewsbury, 2011).

An analysis of several definitions of digital health has shown three distinct applications that are interconnected:

- uses such as monitoring, tracking, and informing health (eg, mobile devices, mobile sensors and wearables, apps, social media);
- enabling health communication among various stakeholders (eg, digital health, virtual consultations); and
- storing, managing, and utilizing health data (eg, electronic medical records, electronic medication systems) (Shaw et al., 2017).

Instruments used in the various areas of digital health present the potential to supply health care workers with an overview of users' past and current health conditions through allowing a review of their health-related information and better communication, independent of location and access (WHO, 2016). Additionally, the implementation of digital technology in medical care could very likely lower turnaround times, resource utilization, medication mistakes, and adverse treatment events; augment the utilization of preventive measures; and enable stronger adherence to clinical recommendations (Keasberry et al., 2017; Nanah and Bayoumi, 2020; Mohsin et al., 2019).

Box 5. Digital Health in Peru

Peru is moving down the path towards implementing the Primary Health Care model with the Ministry of Health (MoH) pioneering this major shift. Digital health competency is a key facilitator for the implementation of the "Redes Integradas de Salud" (in english, Health Integrated Networks), that are enabling a user-centered approach, making use of the single-time data collection protocol, prioritizing quality and opportunity. Over a single year alone, 26 primary public medical institutions were set up with the Electronic Health Records System (developed in-house), making it possible to book appointments across the network via on-line access, smartphones and other digital devices. This year, the MoH additionally set off the Telehealth National Network comprising 198 public medical care facilities linked all over the nation, translating into significant expenditure savings on user transfers by making use of local medical solutions.

Chile and Peru will collaborate to make optimal use of the advantages that information and communications technologies (ICTs) are able to provide for a wide range of public health initiatives. By way of a collective digital project backed up by the Pan American Health Organization and the World Health Organization (PAHO/WHO), both nations will bring forth their experience with ICT techniques, methodologies, and implementation in the medical field, and in this way establish their leadership in developing digital health competency nation-wide. The Chilean and Peruvian ministries of health have publicly expressed strong interest in implementing innovative digital modalities to the medical services accessible to their peoples. Supported by the PAHO/WHO, the ministries will collaborate to facilitate the seeding and growth of initiatives, promoting and strengthening the impact of those initiatives that have the most significant impact, as well as creating a learning environment.

For the duration of approximately one year, the dual country project will aim to promote the sustainable development of Chile's and Peru's medical systems, and to facilitate access to, as well as the quality of, their medical care via the use of ICTs. Moreover, the collaboration is an answer to the third strategic area of the PAHO/WHO eHealth Strategy and Plan of Action, with the objective to "promote and facilitate horizontal cooperation among countries for development of a digital health agenda for the Region."

With the objective of shifting their health systems towards a more people-centered model, some countries see the huge potential of information and digital technologies to make this a reality. Nevertheless, said changes also represent significant challenges for policy makers. Over the past few decades digital technology has modified whole societies as well as the economy worldwide. These changes may be comparable to previous transformations during the industrial revolution. Now, at a point of time of two decades into the 21st century, the medical field is only just experiencing a similar transformation.

Achieving a digital transformation in the medical field is no longer limited by a need to develop the necessary technology – smartphones, mobile apps and other software. The technology is already here. Now, nations must regulate technology in order to foster public service. In addition to regulatory affairs, an overhaul of the structures, policies and institutions that govern health systems is warranted, as is a significant and constant investment in human and institutional capacity building. A true digital transformation is often a political choice.

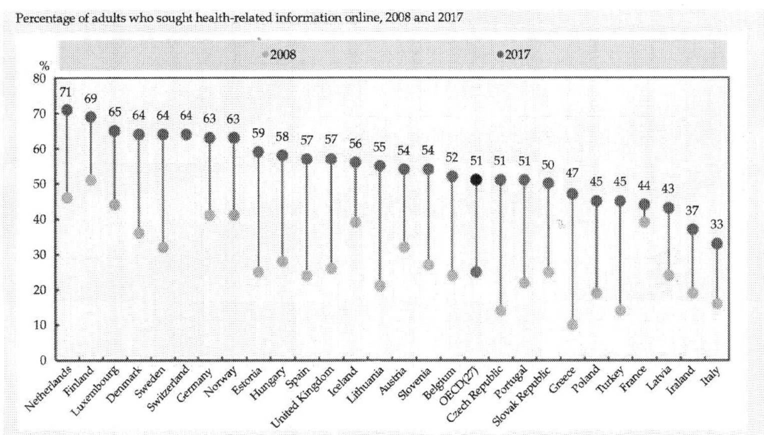

Figure 5. Proportion of adults seeking health information online.

Source: OECD, 2020

Box 6. Digital Health in Ethiopia

Ethiopia remains classified as a low-income country according to the World Bank, as of 2020. Approximately 50% of the country's population lives below the international poverty line. Humanitarian assistance was required by about 18% in 2021. These statistics are partially due to recent hardships including drought, internal conflict and the COVID-19 pandemic.

Currently, life expectancy in Ethiopia is 66.24 years at birth, far below the global average of 72.6 years. This is mostly due to the "severe underfunding of the medical sector," with an unsuitable amount of care facilities, unsuitable delivery of healthcare supplies and significant obstacles when it comes to providing accessible health services to those living in pastoral areas.

Because 79% of Ethiopians reside in rural areas, this represents a significant challenge. In addition, over half of the population is required to walk over 10 kilometers to arrive at the nearest medical care facility. This translates into many Ethiopians going untreated for conditions including malaria, tuberculosis, meningitis and COVID-19. The development of digital health care in Ethiopia will very likely aid in the mitigation of health inequalities between rural and urban areas. Further, it could expand the coverage of health care to those at risk.

The Digital Health Innovation and Learning Center (DHILC), first of its kind, was launched by the Ethiopian Ministry of Health (MoH) in 2020 in Addis Ababa. The DHILC will be a location where medical care professionals are able to design and validate digital health tools, synthesize and promote best practices, and scale-up innovations. The DHILC was built by the MoH with work from the Saint Peter's Specialized Hospital and JSI Research & Training Institute, Inc. via the Ethiopia Data Use Partnership (DUP), supported by the Bill & Melinda Gates Foundation.

The DHILC is a place for both MoH employees and external partners to collaborate and will provide accredited certificate-level education. DHILC will feature a software development and testing environment from the setoff and will serve as a clearinghouse for new digital health solutions that will be applied in the medical care system.

The center is also a place where health care providers can look for and obtain technical and professional backup to address health system implementation challenges. Learning from the experiences of other nations, the DHILC is predicted to address approximately 85% of patients' minor health information system-related problems.

The DHILC has five important functional sections:

1. Data Use Innovation Concept room for collaborative problem-solving and design.
2. eHealth application development and testing room for collaborative eHealth application design, development, and testing.
3. Capacity-building center with two training rooms to hold various digital health applications and data use-capacity-building sessions, including a DHIS2 academy.
4. Resource center where staff and researchers can access electronic scientific publications and other gray literature about Ethiopian health information systems.
5. eHealth support call center to provide remote support to users on eHealth applications and consultations on data quality and use issues.

Ethiopia implemented its first Health Transformation Strategic Plan in 2015 to continue on the significant gains in improving its population's health outcomes. A key point of the plan is the realization of innovation in data-driven medical care by developing and implementing interoperable health information systems that are owned and led by the government.

The need for an international standard on health data governance

Health information is required to improve the quality, safety and user-centered delivery of services, to further scientific innovation, the discovery and evaluation of novel treatments and to redesign and evaluate new models for the delivery of health services. The amount of individual medical information in digital form is already vast, and it is growing with technological developments including digital health and administrative records; behavioral and environmental monitoring devices and apps; and bio-banking and genomic technologies. The scale, capabilities and methodologies of medical information collection, aggregation and analysis are additionally radically dynamic.

When individual medical information is connected and analyzed, an exponential value in information is achieved which can be used to serve the public interest, including more accurate diagnosis, particularly for rare conditions; pinpointing best responders to treatment and tailoring management protocols for optimal outcomes; discovering unsafe practices and treatment options; championing high quality and efficient practices; catching fraud and waste in the system; evaluating the long-term effects of health treatments; and discovering and assessing new health care treatments and practices. Emerging technologies including Big Data analytics, for example, can use enhanced computing power to process wide ranges of data in real time that, when applied, can improve user-care and further the discovery of disease markers and condition-specific treatment.

Nevertheless, information is often held in silos by the institutions collecting them and there are questions on how the potential gains of new analytic techniques can be achieved while guaranteeing the implementation of current information protection standards. A 2013 OECD study reported that many OECD Member States do not have a co-ordinated public policy framework to orient health information utilization and data exchange practices, so as to ensure privacy, facilitate efficiencies, optimize quality and foster innovative research.

There are gains and setbacks from medical information processing at both the personal and community levels. The upkeep of a private health care system is key to effective personal care and management, and to public health. Suitable reconciliation of these risks and gains is required to optimally benefit both single users and the public sector as a whole. Moreover, global collaboration is key to enable countries to safely benefit from health data and to support the production of multi-country statistics, research and other health-related uses of those data that serve the public interest.

For the next half decade ahead, the Health Committee and the Committee on Digital Economy Policy of the OECD will keep coming up with suitable instruments to support the application and dissemination of the recommendation as described below.

The recommendation for the future on-going development of digital health competency are as follows:

1) The interoperability of health data and data analytics must be augmented;
2) More impactful harmonization of health information governance frameworks for cross-country collaboration including the sharing and use of health information must be achieved;
3) Exchange of experiences and best practices in health information security as an answer to the increasing occurrence of malicious attacks on health information must be enhanced.

Digital Health Literacy

In tandem with the digitization of medical care and health services, along with the ranging availability of on-line applications, a wide set of skills is needed to make optimal use of such tools; these skills are called digital health literacy. Health management is evolving in the direction of ever growing user intervention, with the end objective of beneficiaries being able to better manage themselves. This in turn creates the need for better comprehension of health-related competencies that users require in order to optimally handle information and play an active role in managing their health. Health literacy is one of the prime ways in which to achieve this. A definition from 1998 says: "Health literacy represents the cognitive and social skills which determine the motivation and ability of individuals to gain access to, understand, and use information in ways which promote and maintain good health" (Nutbeam, 1998).

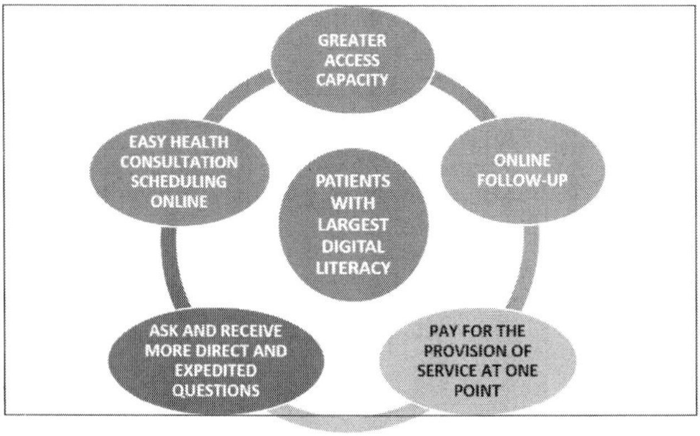

Figure 6. What patients with greater digital literacy want.

Source: Patient Safety and Quality Healthcare. PSQH.com, 2022

According to the above definition, health literacy is limited to oportune tracking of health literacy targeted at a user's ability to read and comprehend health information (Parker et al.,1995; Murphy et al., 1993). This slightly limiting definition has been stretched in later multi component definitions of health literacy to cover, for example, taxonomic levels, navigation in health systems, and social interaction (Osborne et al., 2013; Sørensen et al., 2012; Ishikawa, 2008). Examples of multi component tools for measuring health literacy include the European Health Literacy Survey (HLS-EU) and Health Literacy Questionnaire (HLQ) (Osborne et al., 2013; Sørensen et al., 2012).

In coordination with the growth of health literacy, greater technology use has led to the definition of computer literacy or digital literacy as the understanding of necessary skills in technology use and problem-solving (Gilster, 1997). Digital literacy soon became relevant in the medical field with the sprouting of user-focused digital health care services, for example, email communication with general practitioners and the search for health information online.

In 2006, Norman and Skinner faced this new challenge of understanding the patients' digital health competencies. At the time, they defined electronic health (eHealth) literacy as "the ability to seek, find, understand, and appraise health information from electronic sources and apply the knowledge gained to addressing or solving a health problem" (Norman and Skinner, 2006) and introduced the 8-item eHealth Literacy Scale (eHEALS) instrument for measuring eHealth literacy (Norman and Skinner, 2006). According to the researchers, a patient's eHealth literacy consists of 3 contextual literacies (health literacy, computer literacy, and science literacy) and 3 analytical literacies (traditional literacy, information literacy, and media literacy) (Norman and Skinner, 2006). This model is known as the Lily Model, and it represents the initial understanding of the digital health literacy concept. The model was expanded in 2009 by Chan and Kaufman, who suggested the addition of taxonomic levels for each of the 6 sub literacies, with additional expansions suggested by Gilstad in 2014 adding contextual, cultural, and social dimensions (Chan et al., 2009; Chan and Kaufman 2011; Gilstad, 2014). Moreover, Gilstad proposed a new definition: "eHealth literacy is the ability to identify and define a health problem, to communicate, seek, understand, appraise and apply eHealth information and welfare technologies in the cultural, social and situational frame and to use the knowledge critically in order to solve the health problem" (Gilstad, 2014).

Both Chan and Kaufman, and Gilstad elaborated on the existing concept of eHealth literacy by expanding the Lily model. Nevertheless in 2015, two new conceptual understandings of eHealth literacy came to light.

Box 7. European Health Literacy Survey

Health literacy concerns the capacities of people to meet the complex demands of health in modern society. In spite of the growing attention for the concept among European health policymakers, researchers and practitioners, information about the status of health literacy in Europe remains scarce. The European health literacy survey (HLS-EU) was conducted in eight countries: Austria, Bulgaria, Germany, Greece, Ireland, the Netherlands, Poland and Spain (n = 1000 per country, n = 8000 total sample). The HLS-EU-Q constructed four levels of health literacy: insufficient, problematic, sufficient and excellent. At least 1 in 10 (12%) respondents showed insufficient health literacy and almost 1 in 2 (47%) had limited (insufficient or problematic) health literacy. However, the distribution of levels differed substantially across countries (29–62%). Subgroups within the population, defined by financial deprivation, low social status, low education or old age, had higher proportions of people with limited health literacy, suggesting the presence of a social gradient.Limited health literacy represents an important challenge for health policies and practices across Europe, but to a different degree for different countries. The social gradient in health literacy must be taken into account when developing public health strategies to improve health equity in Europe.

The HLS-EU project is the first study to provide population data on health literacy at the EU level and to enable a comparison of health literacy levels between selected member states. It used a standard survey questionnaire based on a comprehensive conceptual and logic model, applied Eurobarometer standards and ensured consistency in data collection by using one European-wide represented agency.

Whereas the results indicate that more than 10% of the total surveyed population had an inadequate level of health literacy, this proportion varied between 1.8 and 26.9% by country. In turn, almost one in two citizens was affected when considering the proportion of limited health literacy (which varied between 29 and 62%). The considerable proportions of people with limited or inadequate health literacy imply that the health literacy deficit is a challenge for public health in European countries. Moreover, across countries, specific subgroups of the population have a higher proportion of people with limited health literacy than the general population, suggesting the existence of specific vulnerable groups, in addition to the presence of a social gradient in health literacy that is also confirmed by the survey results. Financial deprivation is the strongest predictor of low health literacy, followed by social status, education and age; whereas gender has a minor effect. As such, the HLS-EU data extends the well-documented phenomenon of a social gradient for health and for literacy. Given the richness of the HLS-EU data set, a much more detailed analysis is possible and is partly already being undertaken at both the national and comparative levels.

From the proposed definition arising from the results of the HLS-EU, a systematic clustering of keywords search was carried out by Bautista with the aim of investigating further into definitions of health literacy, digital literacy, and eHealth literacy (Sørensen et al., 2012; Bautista, 2015). This resulted in a new suggestion for a definition of eHealth literacy: "eHealth literacy involves the interplay of individual and social factors in the use of digital technologies to search, acquire, comprehend, appraise, communicate and apply health information in all contexts of health care with the goal of maintaining or improving the quality of life throughout the lifespan" (Bautista, 2015). Simultaneously, the authors of this study, in collaboration with a group of scientists from Deakin University, introduced the eHealth Literacy Framework (eHLF) (Adellund, 2016).

eHLF is comprised of the following 7 dimensions prioritized from a structured process of concept mapping covering both professionals and patients:

- "ability to process information,"
- "engagement in own health,"
- "ability to actively engage with digital services,"

- “feel safe and in control,”
- “motivated to engage with digital services,”
- “access to digital services that work,” and
- “digital services that suit individual needs,”

In combination making up a multi-component definition of eHealth literacy (Norgaard 2015). Based on these, the eHealth Literacy Questionnaire (eHLQ) was created as a tool to measure eHealth literacy based on the 7 dimensions listed above (Abdellund 2016; Kayser et al., 2018).

Measuring Digital Health Competencies

Over the last decades, the healthcare field has experienced rapid changes, with information available online, in addition to mobile applications playing a key role in health care. In tandem with these adaptations, the ability to search, select, appraise, and apply health information from web sources and health care-related digital applications have become ever more impactful for health care users. The combination of said skills are collectively referred to as digital health competency (TNS Political and Social, 2014), or eHealth competency (Norman and Skinner, 200). The relevance of this form of competency is reported in recent studies, demonstrating that patient’s self-perceived skills to utilize information found online has an effect of their health and the quality of their health management, and that insufficient levels of these skills may cause negative outcomes (Hsu et al., 2014; Neter et al., 2012). Hsu et al. (Hsu et al., 2014) reported that digital health competency is linked to various forms of health behavior, such as healthy eating, exercise, and sleeping patterns. Neter and Brainin (Neter and Brainin, 2012) discovered connections between digital health competency and the presence of chronic illness, perceived self-management skills, and more effective comprehension of health status, symptoms, and treatment alternatives.

The existence of a relevant measurement tool for digital health competency is paramount to investigate the effects of these skills, both at a personal level and at a community level. At a personal level—as an example, in routine clinical practice—a measurement instrument may provide backup in making decisions regarding the extent to which a person is able to benefit from specific digital health tools and interventions (Chang et al., 2004; Chan and Kaufman, 2011). Additionally, it could facilitate input to educate patients who require assistance in using internet-based health tools (Xie, 2011; Car et al., 2011). At a community level, a suitable measurement tool could facilitate insight into subgroups at greater risk due to the digitization of implementing unaccessible digital health tools. As an example, past research has reported that digital health competency is linked to socio demographic indicators including age, education, and income (Nater and Brainin, 2012; Chung and Nahm, 2015; Chesser et al., 2016), at the same time that research has demonstrated that certain people lack the skills and knowledge to use internet-based health instruments for their own benefit and might thus even become vulnerable (Chang et al., 2004; Chesser et al., 2016). More detailed information regarding people at risk of low digital health competency can lead to development and personalization of health technologies for these specific populations (Chang et al., 2004; Botts and Horan, 2008).

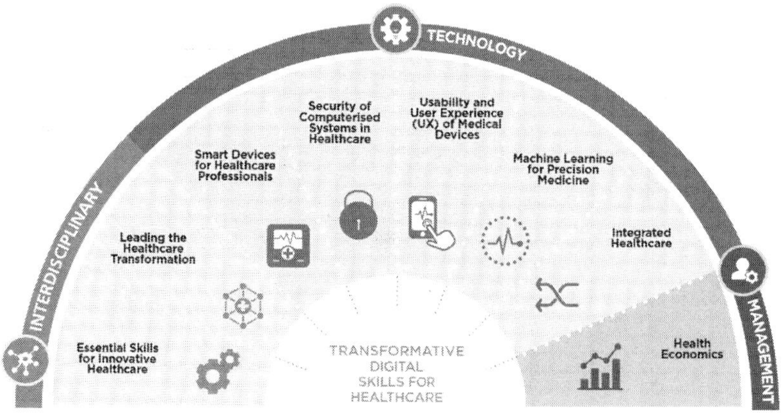

Figure 7. Transformative Digital Skills for Healthcare.

Source: Fraunhofer Institute, 2022

When being investigated, the main aspect in regards to digital health competency has mostly been on the access and utilization of health information that is accessible online (referred to as Health 1.0 applications). However, eHealth is a wide ranging concept that reaches well beyond the simple access to information alone. More current applications (so called Health 2.0 applications) provide all types of interactive technologies, which provide backup for people to exchange information regarding their health (with other users and with health care providers; for example, by way of forums or remote consulting), to self-manage their health (for example, through patient portals), and also to obtain treatment using the Internet (for example, online cognitive behavioral therapy) (van de Belt et al., 2010). In order to determine an individual's ability to utilize this wide range of applications, an evaluation of very diverging skills is required, because making use of interactive Health 2.0 applications requires a different set of skills from simply retrieving health information (Chan and Kaufman, 2011; Norgaard et al., 2015; van Deursen and van Dijk 2011; Norman, 2011).

Research on the digital health competency of patients with rheumatic diseases reported that 6 types of competencies are basic to make suitable use of both Health 1.0 and Health 2.0 applications (van der Vaart et al., 2013). To begin with, individuals require operational and navigation skills to operate a computer and Internet browser; this requires, for example, employing a keyboard, touch screen, and search engine and being able to navigate the Internet. Next, they require information and evaluation skills to search, appraise, and apply information from the Web; this includes, for example, coming up with a suitable search question, selecting reliable search results, comprehension of the obtained results from the search, and being capable of selecting the results that are most reliable and applicable. To use Health 2.0 applications, users require extra skills linked to interactivity on the Internet. This covers contributing with self-generated content to the Internet (for example being able to express oneself in written language) and considering both self and others' privacy (for example understanding who is able to read what one has posted) (Norman, 2011; van der Vaart et al., 2013). Thus, when evaluating an individual's digital health competency, the ability to interact on the Internet should also be taken into account.

The majority of research carried out until now on digital health competency has used the 8-item eHealth Literacy Scale (eHEALS) (Norman and Skinner, 2006), since this has been the only validated tool on the corresponding skills available. The instrument allows for reliable insight into the self-reported competencies of health care users who search and use health information from the Internet. Reports on its validation have demonstrated that it evaluates one overall concept (Norman and Skinner, 2006; van der Vaart et al., 2011), or two separate concepts:searching for and appraising online information (Soellner et al., 2014; Neter et al., 2015). So as to expand the evaluation of digital health competency and to evaluate the broad spectrum of skills that are involved, a new tool has been proposed.

The Digital Health Literacy Instrument (DHLI) has the objective of incorporating the wide range of skills to use both Health 1.0 and Health 2.0 tools (van Deursen AJ, van Dijk, 2011; van der Vaart et al., 2013). To facilitate a more successful evaluation of health competency skills, measurement is done via self-reporting protocols of health care users' perceived skills.

However, it is widely accepted that self-reported information may be biased, because people have the tendency to over- or underestimate their own Internet skills (van der Vaart et al., 2013; Merritt et al., 2005; van Vliet et al., 1994). Research on the validity of the eHEALS predictions has demonstrated that the link between user's own perceived skills and their real performance on Web-based health-related evaluations is minimal (van der Vaart et al., 2011).

The Global Digital Health Index (GDHI) is an interactive digital instrument that tracks, monitors, and measures the use of digital technology for health at an international level. GDHI uses seven key indicator categories to track developments in the process of digitization of health. The components of the GDHI are shown in Figure X below.

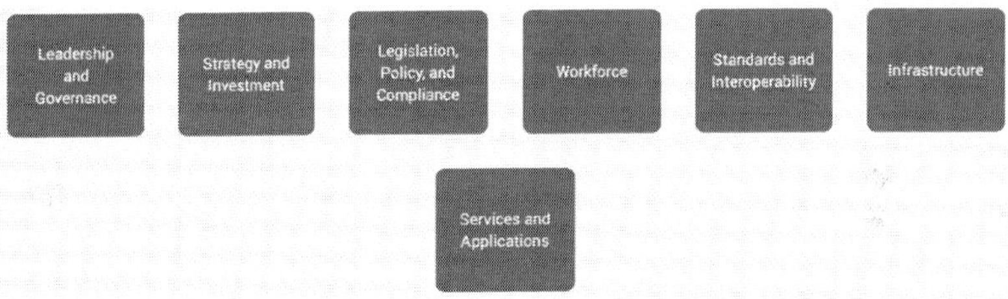

Figure 8. Components of the Global Digital Health Index.

Source: Health Data Collaborative, 2022

Making optimal use of technologies including mobile phones, tablets, remote patient monitoring devices, and sensors as part of the health systems can help save lives, expand the reach of healthcare provided, and lower healthcare costs – nevertheless, numerous countries experience on-going difficulties in setting up and growing sustainable digital health solutions.

At the beginning of 2016, HealthEnabled and the Global Development Incubator (GDI) partnered with Dalberg's Design Impact Group (DIG), ThoughtWorks, and representatives from over 20 countries and over 50 global agencies and organizations to develop the Global Digital Health Index (GDHI), an instrument to assist nations benchmark and track their investments in digital health. Using the World Health Organization (WHO) and International Telecommunications Union (ITU) eHealth Strategy Toolkit, the GDHI is an interactive digital tool that tracks, monitors, and measures the use of digital technology internationally in the various areas of health.

The GDHI has three key goals:

- EMPOWER: The GDHI allows for a visual peek at the status and past development of key performance indicators in digital health at a national and international level. It strengthens health ministries, funders, policy makers, and industry players to make more intelligent and informed decisions for strategic progress regarding how and where to allocate resources.
- EVALUATE: The GDHI compares countries with standardized digital health criteria. It measures the presence and quality of national policies and strategies, risk of investment, and reach of main digital health platforms while giving nations a roadmap for progressive development.
- MOTIVATE: The GDHI aids nations in evaluating their progress and spotting weaknesses within their initiatives in digital health. It provides an incentive for improvement in national digital health systems and more targeted investments internationally.

Regardless of the rapidly growing number of interventions making use of mobile devices that champion the education and self-management of users with chronic conditions, the application of digital health has been rather minimal (Lee et al., 2018; Mahmood et al., 2019). The challenges to applying digital health include missing interest and lack of familiarity with technology, minimal experience with user interaction, and insufficient skills linked to digital health (Agrawal et al., 2019; Dunn and Conard, 2018). Non-users showed less technology-related health competency, more concerns regarding data security, and lower perceived value of utilizing an app when in comparison to users (Price et al., 2017). A pragmatic test of a mobile app for self-management of diabetes demonstrated that only 18.2% of users opened the app regularly during the research period (with a duration of 182 days). During the studyl, approximately 50% of the participants used the app for 10 days or less, and users who were older, did not have personal motivation, and perceived minimal beliefs regarding digital health were much less likely to utilize mobile devices (Agrawal et al., 2019). The success of digital therapeutics, currently the most often used form of intervention where mobile devices are utilized, has been demonstrated to depend on age and user skills suitable to manage the technology when undergoing interventions. This phenomena may cause a potential bias in the digital healthcare services offered (Yan et al., 2021).

Digital health literacy (DHL) is the term given to the specific level of skills and abilities required to make use of digital health technology and services (Robins and Dunn, 2019; Harri et al., 2019). While DHL needs several skills and abilities, the vast majority of research to date has considered DHL to be synonym with eHealth literacy, which is "the ability to seek, find, understand, and appraise health information from electronic sources and apply the knowledge gained to addressing or solving a health problem" (van der Vaart and Drossaert, 2017; Kayser et al., 2018; Griebel et al., 2018). Nevertheless, DHL has a broader reach in the context of technology, covering also mobile devices and health information technology (IT), digital health, and personalized medicine. A step further from DHL is Digital Health Competency.

The Dimensions of Digital Health and How They are Measured

Person-Enabled Health

Person-Enabled Health targets the ability of the health system to meet and deliver on personal needs, values and personalized health targets. It highlights the value and key role of connectivity across individuals and their health teams, developing a partnership based on personal requirements and selection. It leverages digital options (including online tools, handheld devices for remote care approaches, or apps that allow for on-demand health and wellness care) to empower people to self-manage their own conditions, all of this by considering unique life circumstances, preferences, health requirements and options of the user.

Person-Enabled Health is assessed in accordance to:

Personalized care delivery is the individualization of care, where users are the main decision-makers in the management of their own conditions. People select the digital instruments and technologies (for example personal digital tools, mobile devices, wearables) that are most suitable to their individual life circumstances and tailored approaches to care.

Proactive risk management targets the delivery of care that proactively singles out risks to health and wellness, alerts individuals and their health teams about the risks and potential approaches to proactively take action to reduce risk and maintain or optimize progress toward health objectives. Proactive care delivery needs a transformational turn from the siloed, disease control approach currently in use, to one where it is possible to integrate services and one that allows the delivery of care in digital settings for tailored delivery of care to single users and entire communities. Proactive delivery of care translates into being able to anticipate and identify people at risk for health loss and deliver a timely intervention to support and strengthen health.

Predictive population health is the term given to health systems where data is moved and shared along with wide analytic tools to monitor the health of a population to anticipate risks (for example gaps in health screening, risks of chronic conditions, risk of medical mistakes), and develop as well as deliver on strategies to manage and lower risks to population groups, targeting health and wellness. Predictive population health has the characteristic of being informed-based with an infrastructure that utilizes digital tools, dashboards, and public reporting strategies to optimize population health outcomes.

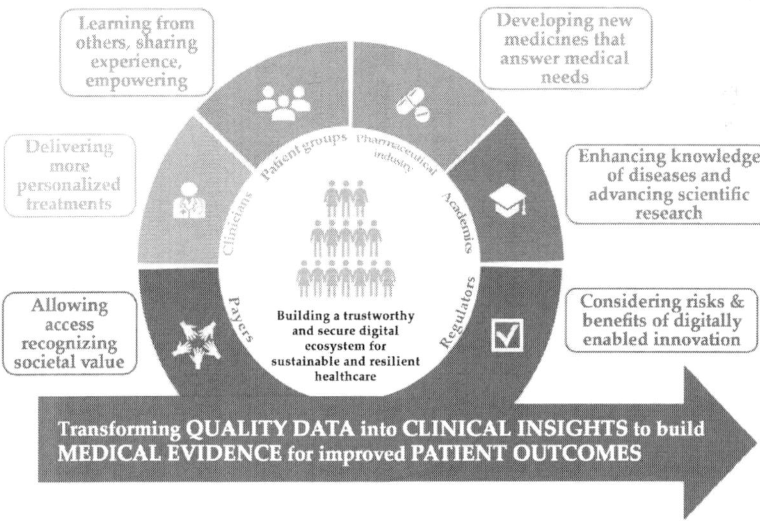

Figure 9. Digital health transformation.

Source: European Federation of Pharmaceutical Industries and Associations, 2022

Person centredness has been discussed across almost if not all fields of health and medicine for several decades, arguing for its value in improving health care. The purpose and proof as to why we should be doing so however is easily taken for granted in general discussion. Clarity, or at least reminding, on why person centredness should be incorporated is crucial to utilizing this effectively. The origin of person centered care was born from the field of psychology half a century ago thanks to Dr Carl Rogers advocating for a shift towards valuing the person's perspective and experience improving success in treatment. The argument for the patient to be respected as an equal partner in health care, notably for decision making, was then discussed as broadly applicable to health and medicine by Tuckett et al in 1985. In the 1990's Wagner and colleagues (1996), as well as Clark et al (1991) explicitly discussed the evidence for improving health outcomes in management of chronic health where the person had been given an active or central role in care planning and delivery. In the same era, the psychologist Albert Bandura who initially specialized in social theories of behavior change (1992) found prominence in health psychology where the field of self-efficacy in relation to improving health outcomes (Bandura, 1992) was now supported by the counter movement from medical researchers. Chronic health by definition requires management over a sustained amount of time and as such is most dependent on the person to be involved in maintaining health and care activities where the physician can only be present and in control for a minority of the disease journey. The inclusion, and arguably, promotion of the patient to a person, especially in chronic health, in increasing levels of control for their health and care journey was now well established and understood to be inherent to allowing the person to be actively involved and in parts responsible for their outcomes. The fundamental purpose of person centered care is therefore one of improving outcomes that can only be achieved with shared control and responsibility rather than simply respecting the person present.

The Digital Health Skills Gap

With the role of technology as a strength force in health system resilience becoming ever more defined, healthcare stakeholders encounter many challenges, including staff with insufficient experience with digital health technologies, limiting their ability to move forward with the digital transformation and future plans.

Increasing healthcare costs, insufficient experienced workers, and employee shortages are creating demand for digital health technologies that are able to improve efficiency of care. This is particularly the case in Australia where border controls have created greater strain on healthcare facilities that were previously dependent on international workers while already at a breaking point from staff shortages. Additionally, the WHO predicts that by 2035 there will be a global shortage of approximately 12.9 million skilled professionals across the healthcare sector, with additional predictions reporting the need for 6 million additional nurses to address international health goals.

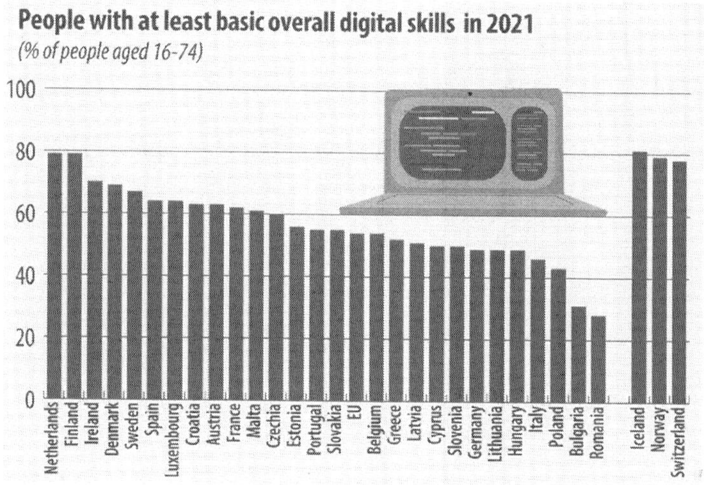

Figure 10. Digital Skill Gap in Europe 2021.

Source: Eurostat, 2021

A point in favor of digital health solutions is that it allows for scalability and adaptation of a network; permitting healthcare staff to continuously grow and improve their technical offering and as an outcome, come up with improved strategies for the management of health based on diverse solutions.

This ongoing capacity to evolve the healthcare model by making use of technology must be met with the corresponding agile education setup, one which is able to keep up with the dynamism. In order for this to take place, there must be ongoing alignment with the stakeholders of health services as well as with clinicians to develop a learning environment that foresees the upcoming requirements of the industry.

Educational institutions and adjoining organizations play an additional proactive role in strengthening education standards collaborations between public and private institutions. This kind of partnership is essential to the development of an effective developmental strategy for healthcare and is a shared opinion by healthcare stakeholders across many countries, with many voicing the opinion that prioritizing strategic collaboration is among the most pressing actions that their institutions currently require so as to successfully implement digital health technologies.

For the purpose of knowledge sharing, collaboration opportunities expand to universities and healthcare technology companies. Private institutions play a decisive role in not only pushing digital development within the healthcare field but in championing the transition as an outcome of their solutions, products and services. This kind of partnership is able to pinpoint key trends and develop a stronger education strategy that answers to the new ways of delivering care. Supported by both the private and public sectors, countries are able to modify care delivery as a national level and adapt the healthcare narrative through the adoption of digital tools.

Box 8. What are basic digital skills?

Examples of data literacy skills include finding information online about goods or services or reading online newspapers, Eurostat explains.

Communication and collaboration skills include sending and receiving emails and using social media. Digital content creation skills include using word processing or spreadsheet software and editing photos, video or audio files.

Safety skills relate to things like limiting access to profile or content on social media sites and changing internet browser settings.

Problem solving skills include selling online, internet banking and installing software or apps.

At 79% each, the Netherlands and Finland score the highest on basic overall digital skills. Ireland is next, with 70%.

Romania, Bulgaria and Poland show the lowest share of basic overall digital skills, at 28%, 31% and 43% respectively.

Eurostat says digital skills are a key indicator in the European Commission'sDigital Decade initiative. This outlines the EU's vision for digital transformation by 2030. Goals include at least 80% of EU citizens aged between 16 to 74 having at least basic digital skills by 2030.

The Role of Software in Digital Health Competencies

Software has been permeating and transforming virtually every industry—including health care-over the last decade.

The software types that drive disruptors in the market, including smartphones, social media, and the sharing economy, have greatly modified the way people live, work, and play. Software is also driving game-changing developments in medicine, including 3D printing, diagnostics at point-of-care, robotics, bioinformatics, synthetic biology, and genomics, but to name a few.

The implementation of software is modifying how clinicians practice medicine, how users manage their own health, and how these two groups interact. Software that is able to perform complex medical functions has been a revolutionary development in digital health technology. This is referred to as software as a medical device (SaMD). SaMD is able to diagnose conditions, suggest treatments, and inform clinical management.

SaMD	Not SaMD
Software that can determine the proper drug dose for a patient, given personalized patient data	Software that operates a pacemaker
Software that can detect and diagnose a stroke by analyzing MRI images	Software that drives or controls an infusion pump's motors
Software that can track the size of a mole over time and determine the risk of melanoma	Electronic health record (EHR) systems
Software that draws on data from other digital devices to determine risk factors associated with epileptic seizures	Software in the machines that assemble medical devices

Source: Deloitte Analysis

Additionally, not all health software is regulated by the FDA; such applications are considered outside this paper's scope. According to draft FDA guidance released in December 2017, "Changes to Existing Medical Software Policies Resulting from Section 3060 of the 21st Century Cures Act"[2] and "Clinical and Patient Decision Support Software,"[3] general wellness applications, such as those that track heart rate and exercise routines, are not subject to FDA review. Neither is lower-risk decision support software that allows the health care provider, caregiver, or patient to independently review the basis of a treatment recommendation. A hypothetical application that provides recommendations for insulin dosage based on blood sugar level readings, for example, would not be subject to FDA review, so long as the recommendations are consistent with FDA-approved labeling for the insulin.

Figure 11. What is and is not SaMD.

Source: medable.com, 2022

The International Medical Device Regulators Forum (IMDRF), of which the US Food and Drug Administration (FDA) is a member, describes SaMD as software that is able to work on general-purpose (non-medical) computing platforms; can be employed in tandem with other products such as medical devices; and can interface with other medical devices or other general-purpose hardware and software that give input to SaMD.

Software that is essential for hardware to function—for example, software that helps an MRI's magnets turn or animates an X-ray control panel—is not considered SaMD. Nor is software that is limited to retrieving information, organizing data, or optimizing processes.

SaMD is able to offer countless benefits in the health field. A key one is that it allows users to play a more involved role in their own health management. As an example, WellDoc's BlueStar tracks blood-glucose information and provides individualized coaching to facilitate management of treatment and medication among diabetic patients.

Box 9. WellDoc Blue Star

WellDoc Blue Star is a singular, connected, whole-person care platform that can address complex combinations of the world's most widespread conditions and co-morbidities.

The Welldoc platform offers:

- Support for multiple chronic conditions
- A total ecosystem solution
- AI with a higher IQ

The Welldoc platform supports type 1 and type 2 diabetes, hypertension, heart failure and prediabetes, with behavioral health insights. Their approach addresses cardio-metabolic conditions, tailored to an individual's specific combination of condition all intended to bring more meaningful digital engagement and health support.

Welldoc's secure platform scales care management programs for a whole-person view that helps deliver coordinated care and meaningful interventions at the right time.

Often powered by artificial intelligence (AI)-enabled algorithms, some SaMD is also able to more accurately diagnose a condition when compared to trained clinicians. In the United Kingdom, the National Health Service (NHS) is collaborating with Google's DeepMind to allow physicians to spot timely signs of sight-threatening eye diseases. Google's UK-based AI division will employ machine learning to analyze over one million anonymous eye scans, creating computer algorithms that are able to detect early warning signs that doctors—including highly experienced ones—might miss. The idea is that this partnership may allow for earlier detection and management of common eye diseases including age-related macular degeneration and diabetic retinopathy, the latter being the fastest-growing cause of blindness globally.

Box 10. DeepMind

DeepMind is a division of Alphabet, Inc. responsible for developing general-purpose artificial intelligence (AGI) technology. That technology is also known as Google DeepMind. DeepMind uses raw pixel data as input and learns from experience.

DeepMind has created a neural network that learns how to play video games in a fashion similar to that of humans, as well as a Neural Turing machine, or a neural network that may be able to access an external memory like a conventional Turing machine, resulting in a computer that mimics the short-term memory of the human brain.

DeepMind made headlines in 2016 after its AlphaGo program beat a human professional Go player Lee Sedol, a world champion, in a five-game match, which was the subject of a documentary film. A more general program, AlphaZero, beat the most powerful programs playing go, chess and shogi (Japanese chess) after a few days of play against itself using reinforcement learning. In 2020, DeepMind made significant advances in the problem of protein folding with AlphaFold. In July 2022, it was announced that over 200 million predicted protein structures, representing virtually all known proteins, would be released on the AlphaFold database. DeepMind posted a blog post on 28 April 2022 on a single visual language model (VLM) named Flamingo that can accurately describe a picture of something with just a few training images.[16][17] In July 2022, DeepMind announced the development of DeepNash, a model-free multi-agent reinforcement learning system capable of playing the board game Stratego at the level of a human expert.

In the past, the FDA has regulated SaMD in the same way as hardware-based medical devices. Nevertheless, in accordance with the FDA's Digital Health Program, this approach is "not well suited for the faster, iterative design, development, and type of validation used for software-based medical technologies." For example, software developers are able to make continuous, post-launch modifications to their products remotely. These modifications may be linked to security or feature updates, or product alterations based on data from the user.

As another example, the Google DeepMind algorithm may in the near future be able to detect early signs of eye disease as early as six months prior to what a clinician is able to do. Since this device is employed on more people, its ability to detect abnormalities is likely to become more precise and sophisticated, permitting even earlier detection—possibly as much as a year before clinicians are able to do so. However, there is a caveat: in order to update the algorithm's functionality, the maker of the device may require a product update to be released, in this way modifying the product that was originally approved by the FDA. The current regulatory process highlights thorough vetting prior to product release into the market, without much continuous following evaluation.

In addition, numerous SaMD developers are software developers who have not previously dealt with the FDA. They may find the regulatory process tough to navigate, which may lead to challenges in bringing products to market and, possibly, dissuade them from developing SaMD offerings to begin with. To champion medical innovation among these developers, the FDA might be required to clarify and simplify the regulatory process.

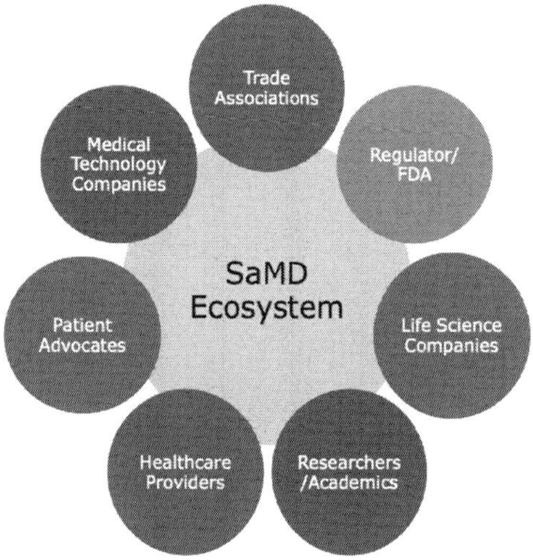

Figure 12. Key players in the software as a medical device (SaMD) system.

Source: othogonal.io, 2022

SaMD is able to continually compile and analyze information on medical images, physiological status (for example, body temperature), biomarker outcomes or any other indicator that the SaMD algorithm processes. This capacity, which is at the center of SaMD, becomes worrisome in terms of cybersecurity and protection of users' information. In December of 2016, the FDA published a guide on cybersecurity in medical devices, yet the potential to compile, analyze, and keep user data has led some advocacy organizations, such as the American Hospital Association, to approach the FDA demanding even greater transparency surrounding information handling and security needs for the protection of user information. By developing a novel regulatory review process where device manufacturers and users are willing to disclose real-world data, it is possible to more effectively track these products as they change and assure that they stay safe and effective.

The significant advancement of digital health technologies poses a clear imperative for a novel regulatory framework that highlights the main differences between these products and traditional medical devices. Creating a process for the effective regulation of SaMD may be the first step to developing a new regulatory paradigm for the whole digital health arena, as well as for other regulated industries in which software has become essential and disruptive.

Box 11. Healthcare and digital care in Australia

In accordance with the Philips Health Index Australian report for 2021, approximately 43% of healthcare leaders consider workforce inexperience with technology as the strongest challenge to experiencing greater adoption of digital solutions. About a third of Australian healthcare leaders would prefer to hire new employees with expertise in digital user data, while a similar number (29%) of leaders mentioned employee shortages as an additional challenge In the Future Health Index report for 2020, focused on the perspectives of the next generation of healthcare professionals and their digital competency, 47% of younger Australian healthcare workers reported they did not know how to use digital user data to optimize patient care.

A key factor of creating an effective digital healthcare ecosystem is addressing the change management needed to ease the transition. This covers not only charting the different management solutions that may be provided virtually and those that must be delivered in-person, but effectively displaying the value of novel forms of working as well as the effect of taking up digital health on the Australian workforce and the merging of technology in providing support for these tasks.

Accounting for 14% of Australian workers, the Australian Government has placed strong interest in guaranteeing the education standards of the Health Care and Social Assistance sector. Both local and national government organizations have a responsibility to champion for and direct the implementation of the education reforms needed to support the transition process of the national healthcare system. In addition, greater investment in education nation-wide has the capacity to reduce ongoing staff shortages, permitting the local healthcare system to develop a workforce of local talent.

This covers outlining novel basic requirements for education in digital health technologies through the optimal collaboration of both the healthcare and education fields. By way of a standardization process, efforts to reduce skills gaps through effective learning formats may be evaluated more holistically and alterations to requirements can be put in place across the board. By taking a blanket approach, Australia's government may ensure that everyone within the sector is empowered to support the future of healthcare, armed with suitable skills.

WORLD HEALTH ORGANIZATION GLOBAL STRATEGY ON DIGITAL HEALTH

Internationally, the World Health Organization is paying greater attention to digital health competency, generally defined as "the ability to seek, find, understand, and appraise health information from electronic sources and apply the knowledge gained to addressing or solving a health problem".

In accordance with this definition, digital health competency seems to exclusively refer to the implementation of digital tools to access general health information. It does not encompass the important point of being literate about digital health. As part of the original definition, WHO covered digital health competency as a component of the Digital Health Ecosystem, in addition to telemedicine, big data and governance interventions. Over the past few years, it has made available relevant documents, including *Digital Technologies: Shaping the Future of Primary Health Care* (2018) and the first *WHO Guideline Recommendations on Digital Interventions for Health System Strengthening (*2019).

The main guiding principles targeted at directing the global strategy in the direction of an appropriate and sustainable adoption of digital health in the context of country-wide health systems and strategies are:

- Acknowledge that institutionalization of digital health in the national health system requires a decision and commitment by countries
- Recognize that successful digital health initiatives require an integrated strategy
- Promote the appropriate use of digital technologies for health
- Recognize the urgent need to address the major impediments faced by least-developed countries implementing digital health technologies

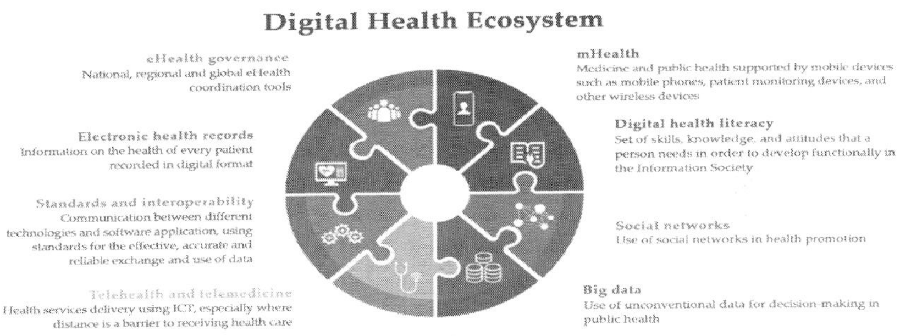

Figure 13. Digital Health Ecosystem.

Source: WHO, 2020

Furthermore, the WHO has put forward a compendium of strategic targets intended to give guidance and coordination on international digital health transformation and to further develop synergies between initiatives and stakeholders to optimize health outcomes and reduce associated risks at all levels. These include:

- Promote international collaboration and advance the knowledge exchange on digital health

This strategic target has the objective of aligning countries and stakeholders to act in conjunction on global opportunities for the improvement of health and work towards universal health coverage, while addressing challenges, identifying and communicating risks, and targeting threats linked to the use of digital technologies both to improve health and to facilitate universal health coverage, the core of the health-related Sustainable Development Goals. This target encourages action on routine opportunities independently of their situation.

- Maximize the impact of both newly developed and existing collaborations and partnerships in the wider digital health ecosystem.

Awareness of and investments in digital health design and implementation are exchanged across domains; thus, this target aims to strengthen collaborations and partnerships with additional agencies within the United Nations, countries and other stakeholders and to assist in building new ones.

- Assess and promote the newest, most suitable and innovative health technologies.

Leading health technologies are developing new and advanced health care services and solutions. This sub-objective aims to ensure that the quality and results of novel health technologies are evaluated in order to allow for their timely adoption and promotion. Norms, standards, policies and regulations are required to secure the investment, sustainability, quality, security and safety of both digital health products and latest health technologies that not only are used in health care but that may also be directly promoted to individuals.

The below listed policy options and actions are suggested:

- co-develop the international strategy on digital health and set mechanisms for strengthening country-wide digital health strategies and set up key collaborations on agreed-upon suitable implementation of digital technologies to reach national health and well-being goals;
- set up a knowledge management system to capture and share good practices, knowledge about implementation of novel methodologies and techniques, evidence and lessons learned on digital health across countries and global communities;

- provide support for countries in setting up information centers for the monitoring of diseases to manage and set off oportune decisions during epidemics and other public health emergencies;
- align countries and stakeholders to collectively address international, regional and national obstacles and opportunities; highlight, manage and communicate risks; and reduce threats linked to the implementation of digital technologies to provide better and universal health coverage.

The below listed outputs are proposed:

- Prioritization is given to digital health and its integration into global, regional and national health systems by way of established bodies and mechanisms for governance;
- Groups of multiple stakeholders are established and meet on a regular basis to steer suitable usage and growth of digital health and innovation in order to speed up the progress towards the health-related Sustainable Development Goals;
- Centers for disease surveillance information collection and analysis are set up or strengthened at national, regional and global levels.

These objectives aim to promote and provide support for each country to own, adapt and strengthen its strategy on digital health in the most suitable form for its vision, context at a national level, health situation and trends, resources made available and guiding values.

Further, they encourage the development of a country-wide strategy on digital health through a multi stakeholder approach made up of actors working within action groups and with the following core components in mind:

(1) leadership
(2) investment
(3) services and scaling up possibilities
(4) sustainability
(5) flexible digital infrastructure
(6) workforces that are adaptable
(7) legislation and compliance
(8) user-centered approach

The above listed strategies should all be created while the necessary alignment of country stakeholders is secured in order that the requirements and expectations with given resources be considered.

In order to ensure the sustainability and growth of digital health, the strategic objective targets a development of cross-sectoral partnerships at national level to align resources and investments. This strategy also looks to work with existing digital health collaborations to push global digital health efforts. Creating national collaborations for the sustainability of digital health development would accelerate their uptake by WHO Member States.

Even though each individual country is expected to review or create and own its strategy from initiation to implementation, these strategic targets aim to set up human and institutional forces for the safe and suitable use and scale-up of digital health by reinforcing the commitment and systematic participation of all stakeholders in each country. The strategy underpins the promotion of innovative integration of digital technologies into health systems.

To reinforce health systems by implementing digital technologies, a main objective is to identify ways for capacity building and create a digitally-capable health workforce. Requirements will vary from one country to the next, but they often include basic capacities, covering leadership and governance, and the creation of a skilled health and technological workforce.

The below listed policy options and actions are suggested:

- provide stimulus for and support every country to take up or review, own, and reinforce its national digital health strategy in a manner that enhances the level of maturity of the country in regards to digital health so as to reach positive health outcomes that align with national health plans, up to date norms and standards as well as universal health coverage;
- ascertain that institutions, stakeholders and staff involved in the provision of health care services and all users are suitably participating in the design and development phases;
- allow for systematic participation of all relevant stakeholders in the achievement of the vision and its strategic objectives as part of a wholistic digital health ecosystem at the country level;
- define a country-wide digital health architecture diagram, adopt open-source health information standards and target reusable systems or assets including interoperability of health information

systems both at country and global levels in order to establish an innovative integration of different digital technologies making use of shared services, ensuring information is of good and comparable quality;

- take up a legal and ethical frameworks for securing user safety, information security, suitable use and ownership of health information, privacy data recoverability, in addition to protection of intellectual property rights;
- highlight and share sustainable financing models in support of digital health development and sharing of learning to develop future products and services. This is particularly key in artificial intelligence such as machine learning, implementation, integration and maintenance, including economic incentives.
- design, implement and track a change management strategy, to support conducive organizational behavior surrounding novel digital health processes and practices.

The following outputs are envisaged:

1) A country-wide digital strategy for digital health or equivalent strategic framework is present, is part of the national health strategy and is actively employed in guiding growth and accelerating development towards the health-related objectives of the Sustainable Development Goals and in the context of digital change of health systems.
2) a changing digital health maturity model evaluation to direct prioritization of national involvement in digital health is created to support primary health care and universal health coverage.

- Fortify governance for digital health at global, regional and national levels

This strategic target covers strengthening the governance of digital health at national and international levels through the making of sustainable and robust governance frameworks and creating the capacity for digital health at international and country levels. Governance for digital health has the objective of strengthening the capabilities and skills required for countries to stimulate, innovate and scale up digital health technologies.

The strategic objective champions standards for safety, security, privacy, interoperability, and the ethical employment of information within and outside the health field. Actions to fortify governance should encompass establishing principles and achieving cross-sectoral and international agreements for information exchange, quality and accuracy of health information and prioritization of investment projects and policy. It should additionally cover principles for the ethical utilization of health information in technologies including artificial intelligence and big data analytics.

In addition, the aim is to improve assessment and monitoring of and research on the application of digital health in the health field. The research plan should cover the need to improve and extensively communicate evidence and information on the utilization of digital health across all levels. Investigation into and evaluation of digital health outcomes and impact are basic to support its safe application, to set up and promote accountability and to justify the financial investment. The plan should also cover the need to stimulate the development and testing of technologies, methodologies and infrastructures that surpass obstacles to the application of digital health to health priorities. This plan is tightly connected to capacity-building of research teams and the improvement and sharing of methods and data analytics.

The following policy options and actions are suggested:

1) fortify governance of digital health at country and global levels by leveraging current structures and as suitable, creating sustainable and robust governance structures, including regulatory frameworks, and the feasibility for the implementation of evidence-based and proven digital health solutions at international and country levels;
2) coordinate investments in evidence-based steps to evaulate, promote and communicate new and innovative health technologies for country-wide scaled digital health programmes using a person-centered approach to drive actions and investments based on informed decisions;
3) promote and facilitate digital health competencies in the education and training programs of all healthcare professionals and allied workers;
4) promote capacity-building for leaders of public health authorities, connected agencies and policy-makers to make information-based decisions to support digital health investments.

The following results are predicted:

1) governance exists, according to the WHO-led creation of regulatory framework, to agree on internationally-suitable utilization of health data and on terms such as health information as a global public good and to define principles of equitable information-sharing principles for research, consistent metadata and definitions, AI and information analytics, and primary and secondary use of information;
2) a voluntary guideline on international interoperability standards for digital health is created in collaboration with decision makers and adopted, that
a) aims to grow upon results already widely achieved,
b) covers a list of commonly agreed use cases for the public health care sector, its functional needs and a set of functional and technical specifications, standards, semantics and profiles derived from it,
c) defines needs for a sound legal and regulatory framework with specifically defined roles for information governance and
d) covers political leadership regarding public investment, procurement and standardization to develop an interoperable digital health ecosystem at the country and global levels;
3) global guidance on planning, development and implementation of digital hospitals, digital clinical trials and digital therapeutics is created;
4) A collection of recommendations is created for pseudonymization and anonymization of health information.

- Champion people-centered health systems facilitated by digital health

This strategic target promoted digital health literacy, gender equality and women's empowerment and inclusive approaches to uptake and manage digital health technologies.

The strategic objective places individuals at the center of digital health through the uptake and utilization of digital health technologies in growing and strengthening health service delivery. The individual is a key component in the delivery of trust-based, people-centered care. This approach encompasses not only patients, families and communities but also the health workers who must be prepared to deploy or utilize digital health technologies as part of their work. Making plans for capacity- building includes workforce evaluation, ranging from professionals in information and communication technologies to healthcare employees giving care services. Due to its intrinsically multidisciplinary and interdisciplinary nature, capacity-building requires instilling capabilities, attitudes and skills which may cover everything from computer sciences, strategic planning, finance and management to health sciences and the delivery of care, depending on the digital health application and its context.

Evaluation of the workforce should also keep in mind the implications for the health labor market of bringing in digital technologies and their management. This aim would require countries to turn away from the current disease focused systems to an integrated approach with the service receiver at its core.

Attitudes towards, practices in and public awareness of digital health must also be covered. Possible actions can cover improving digital health literacy at the population level, engagement of service receivers, families and communities, and education of users regarding health. More efficient responses to the social and commercial determinants of health to better digital health-enabled health systems will require the engagement of civil society but also non-health sectors and actors. Growing awareness of evidence based self-management tools and greater access to these is a further action to keep in mind.

The following policy options and actions are suggested:

1) place individuals at the center of digital health by way of the most suitable health data ownership, adoption and utilization of digital health technologies and development of suitable literacy; the approach will cover not only patients, families and communities but also healthcare professionals and providers;
2) develop processes for health management at the population level by way of digital health applications that shift health and well-being from reactive-care models to active community-based models, and lower the burden of information collection from front-line workers by reorienting reporting-based tools into service delivery tools;
3) set up monitoring and evaluation models to allow for monitoring the contribution of digital systems to health system processes, health workforce processes, and personal and community health needs;

4) fortify gender equality and health equity programs and accessibility for people with disabilities to promote an inclusive digital society with enhanced digital health compctency. When planning and prioritizing digital health programs, relevant points of inequality should be evaluated in order to guarantee that the introduction of digital health technologies does not make these worse and that access for specific population groups is ensured. Furthermore, the clear potential of digital technologies to champion for health equity should be leveraged. With an appropriate design, digital solutions can propel inclusiveness as digital connectivity are able to overcome physical barriers;
5) set up mechanisms for more efficient engagement of the public and transparency in country-wide as well as global digital health decision-making processes, for example through global consultation processes or a stakeholder discussion;
6) create digital health training (Massive Open Online Courses) to build up digital health literacy;
7) create a global communication campaign to sensitize individuals to the benefits of digital health solutions and the utilization of their information for public interest investigations, and thus promote the vision of individuals being actors of innovation.

The following results are predicted:

1) Improved digital health competency in making use of and comprehending digital health technologies and systems in addition to health information is prioritized, and the validated tools are accessible by all people;
2) a framework permitting individual feedback in validating the performance of digital health tools and services, dissemination of increasing digital health demand is set up and utilized;
3) international basic health data standards for prioritized digital health technologies and processes are set up, adopted and applied at country level;
4) International guidance on personalized medicine is created.

Box 12. Digital Health Malaysia

Digital Health Malaysia (DHM), earlier known as Telemedicine Development Group (TDG) was started in 2015. It is a platform where healthcare professionals, researchers and the industry work together to advance the country's digital health programs. In collaboration with relevant ministries and agencies, it regularly collects information from stakeholders of various background and inter-disciplines, interchanges ideas and explores partnership opportunities in the areas of telemedicine, telehealth and AI. It follows the National Science Technology and Innovation (STI) Policy and the ever-changing triple helix ecosystem (Regulator/Researcher/Industry).

DHM connects key players from policy makers, industries, academia, medical practitioners and the medical providers, to drive Malaysia into the information technology arena. It identifies the importance of a good alignment of policy, innovation and research to optimize the impact of and reduce miscommunication and duplication of efforts. It targets a contribution to the country's social and economic development by way of a strategic leadership role in digital health. The Mission of DHM covers the following areas:

- Establishing an inclusive digital healthcare ecosystem ination-wide
- Setting up an expert group to advise, facilitate, regulate and spearhead the uptake of digital health.
- Contributing to the country's economic and social development by way of relevant digital policy, research and creation of innovative digital healthcare solutions.
- Leading and facilitating digital health innovation by way of industry collaboration (open data architecture and standard).
- Establishing an intuitive platform for the design and development of state-of-art, simple and world-class connected healthcare solutions
- Developing into a one stop center for domestic and global digital healthcare stakeholders.
- Establishing a center of excellence for policy, legislation and regulation in digital health.
- Becoming the preferred center for foreign and local stakeholders in digital healthcare solutions.

In addition, four Special Interest Groups have been set up as part of DHM to better serve the members and the industry. These groups include focus on various considerations to be borne when developing a digital health ecosystem and are:

1. Policy & Regulation
2. Knowledge Dissemination / Networking
3. R&D, Clinical Trials
4. Certifications, Go-to Market & Manufacturing

CURRENT DIGITAL HEALTH STATUS IN HIGH INCOME COUNTRIES

The digitalisation of everyday life is a development that has not only been taking place over the past several decades, but has been strongly accelerated by the COVID-19 pandemic. Digitalisation is one of the key processes pushing forth change in the economic, socio-political, and cultural spheres worldwide, in tandem with globalization and demographic modifications (Petersen and Steiner, 2019).

Work, social interactions, health and education services, and recreational activities have been collectively forced to make (further) use of digital technologies and platforms, as the majority of the world transitioned to digital settings at the beginning of the COVID-19 pandemic (Almeida et al., 2020). Nevertheless, not only is greater attention given to digital divides through COVID-19, digital and technological development has neither equally nor equitably crossed all roadblocks of society across the world, further growing the gap between digital divides (Scheerder et al., 2017; Unwin and de Bastion, 2009; van Dijik, 2012). Digital divides are a global challenge and threaten to turn into the new face of inequality because of their potentially detrimental effects on the Sustainable Development Agenda (Honeyman et al., 2020; Hidalgo et al., 2020).

In its Skills Agenda for Europe in 2016, the European Commission first identified the significant requirement for the development of digital skills (European Commission, 2016) as – at the time of writing – approximately half of the European Union's (EU) population was missing basic digital skills, whereas 20% had none at all. This is even more problematic in the context of the rapid progression into the Digital Age arising from the COVID-19 pandemic—specifically the changes in healthcare and public health (European Commission, 2021; Sonnier, 2017; Odonc et al., 2019; van Kessel et al., 2022), yet in addition to greater determinants in health, including ways of working and access to education (scheerder et al., 2017; Sonnier, 2017; Sieck et al., 2021; Cowhey and Aronson, 2017). As an example, it is possible to consider the use of AI-assisted diagnoses and the utilization of telehealth for physical and mental health issues, propelled by the symbiotic necessity to maintain patients out of hospitals where they could have a high risk of spreading or contracting COVID-19 and reducing physical contact with medical workers (Ferdandez et al., 2021). An additional example is the strong role that social media has played in spreading factually inaccurate information throughout the pandemic (Abbas et al., 2021; de Albuquerque et al., 2021; Su et al., 2021).

Digital competency can no longer be considered a luxury; these skills are basic to modern governance, societal and economic functioning, and access to sections of the healthcare and public health systems (Cowhey and Aronson, 2021)—as demonstrated in the European Skills Agenda 2020 update (European Commission, 2020).

While COVID-19 has demonstrated that it is possible to live in a digital society, it emphasized existing health and economic inequalities and increased digital divides across the world (Honeyman et al., 2020). The question thus remains whether the contemporary European ecosystem is capable– let alone suitably ready – to safely and sustainably uphold a digital society.

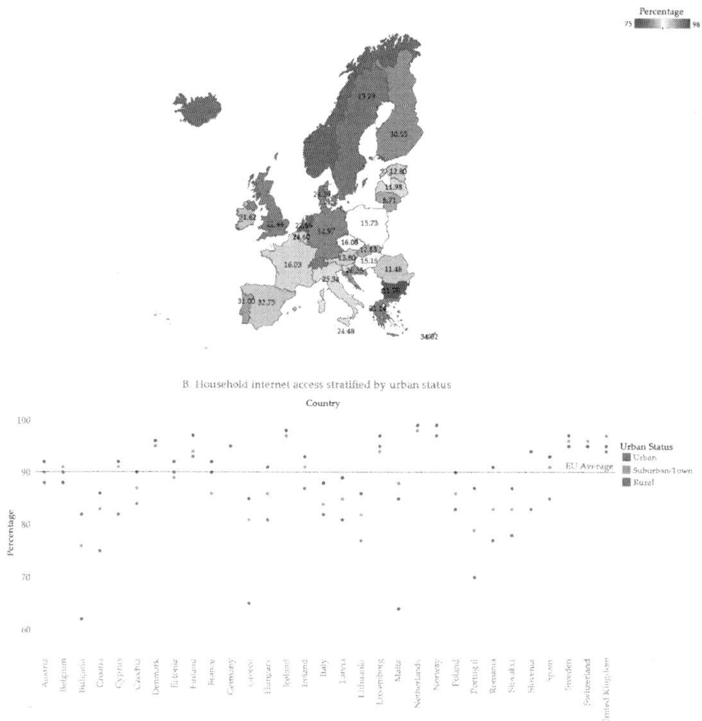

Figure 14. Overall internet access of households in Europe.

Source: Statista, 2019

To further illustrate the question above, the United Kingdom's Office for National Statistics reported in 2019 that about 10% of the adult population did not use the Internet. Additionally, Global Kids Online reported in 2021 that approximately 14% of children under 19 in Europe still did not have frequent internet access (Global Kids Online, 2021; Office of National Statistics Uk, 2019). Nevertheless, these statistics only address the first level of digital divides (binary Internet access), while the second (Internet skills) and third levels (tangible and beneficial outcomes of internet use) remain largely unknown. Demographic characteristics, which are a known influence on the development of digital skills (Scheerder et al., 2017; Kickbusch et al., 2021), have been minimally explored in past investigations.

Previous studies have shown that Europe has an average Internet access rate of 90%, yet fail to specify for different demographics and do not address the presence or lack of digital skills. Young populations, high education levels, employment, and living in an urban environment seem to positively influence the development of higher digital skills.

Box 13. Digital Health in Kuwait: wealth outside the Western World

In Kuwait, the industry for healthcare is approaching a time for digital innovation, as both public and private parties pour resources into their digital transformation. The process, however, remains full of gaps. Several key healthcare institutions have, or are in the process of incorporating innovative digital setups into their activities- mainly in areas including health records, telemedicine, and mobile applications - yet there is currently no connection between institutions. Although a few companies have started taking the necessary strategic and managerial steps needed for the process, the application of a full digital transformation remains piecemeal and short of a national interconnected environment, a required first step to unleashing the full potential of the revolution using advanced technologies including cloud computing and AI.

Across all fields, including healthcare, the Covid-19 pandemic has sped up the digitization process, with remote e-health solutions in particular setting themselves up as clear winners. This translated well for startups related to healthcare in the MENA region, in particular those that offer remote solutions as well as digital services targeting health gravities.

In general, healthcare entrepreneurs have been demonstrating remarkable force and innovation, with startups creating user-centered digital health solutions that leverage state of the art technologies including artificial intelligence and blockchain. Simultaneously, the pandemic has pushed healthcare institutions to reconsider their priorities and strategies: institutions have aimed to allow remote work, lower spending, and speed up the incorporation of digital solutions that augment efficiency. In the future, healthcare organizations will have to deal with the long term impacts of the epidemic, with increasing evidence suggesting that survivors could still face complications for years to come.

Internet access across Europe

Internet access is available to most of the population of Europe (ranging from 75 to 98%). However, there are some geographical differences across regions. The North and North-West are reported to have significantly higher internet access rates in comparison to other European regions (94-98% compared to 89-91% in Central and South-West and 75-87% in South and East). Similarly, urban areas report more consistent levels of internet connectivity when compared to rural regions (82-99% versus 62-99%). Significant differences are reported in rural Southern and Eastern Europe (62-75%) in comparison to urban areas (82-87%). A lower income is also likely to be linked with lower levels of internet access (33-96% compared to 65-100%; 83-100%; and 96-100% for the second, third, and fourth income quartile respectively) (van Kessel et al., 2022).

Digital Skills Across Europe

Most of the strongly digitally skilled people in Europe are found in the Northern and North-Western parts of the continent, demonstrating that over 50% of people possess more than basic digital skills. On the other hand, South-Eastern Europe reports below 20% of people with higher than basic digital skills. This is the opposite in people with minimal digital skills, who are often reported in South-Eastern Europe, while less reported in North-Western Europe.

Considering the data that has been collected thus far, low age can be linked with better developed digital skills, whereas older age is likely to be connected with lesser digital skills. Taking that point into consideration, the development of higher digital skills among younger individuals is inconsistent in Europe as indicated by the reported range (22-85%). Thus, it can be assumed that age requires an interaction with additional factors to reliably produce improved digital skills. The presence of higher digital skills is likely to be reduced with age, whereas reduced digital skills augment with age. Higher than basic digital skills are in the majority found among high education (29-84%), while less so in low education (2-48%). The opposite is true of low digital skills (2-29% and 20-51% respectively). Urban areas demonstrate slightly more consistent higher than basic skills (17-63%) in comparison to rural locations (5-61%), while rural locations report a similar spread of reduced digital skills (13-46%) as urban locations (11-43%). Students and employed people report having the highest proportion of higher than basic digital skills (29-87% and 13-66% respectively). Additionally, high income is linked with the development of stronger digital skills (17-74%), although the wide spread here must also be noted, implying that higher-income levels alone are insufficient.

A positive cross-country correlation between the high capital stock and income/earnings and the digital skills development can be found. In addition, the comparative analysis demonstrates that the cost of access to the internet bears minimal influence on digital literacy levels. These findings are in accordance with the affordability of internet access costs, including their small share within the average income/earnings. This last point means that the influence of the European cross-country capital/income/earnings strata regarding the digital skills development is complex and cannot be limited to internet service pricing only.

Stratification by educational level demonstrates significant differences in higher than basic digital skills in the age category 16-24 (43-96% in high education versus 16-86% in low education). The age groups 25-54 and 55-74 with high education report higher levels of higher than basic skills (34-89% and 13-63% respectively) in comparison to medium and low education (5-55% and 0-46%; and 0-28% and 0-15% respectively). Females with higher education demonstrate reduced levels of higher than basic digital skills (29-82%) in comparison to males (28-87%). For medium and low levels of education, males report higher basic skills (6-56% and 3-55%) more often than females 6-51% and 1-47%). Lower digital skills are underreported in males with medium and low education (14-57% and 18-50%) in relation to females (17-53% and 18-57%).

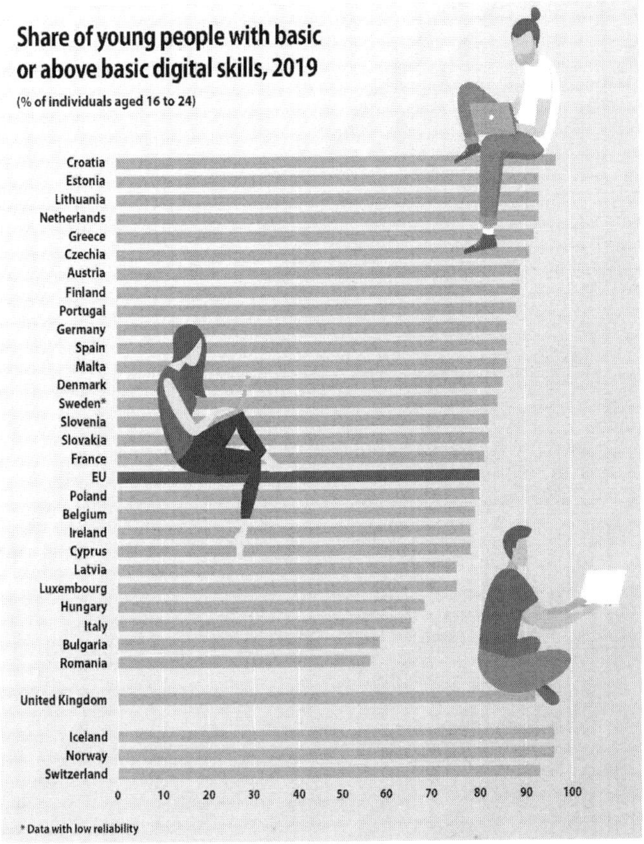

Figure 15. Share of individuals (aged 16-74) with above basic digital skills in 2019.

Source: Eurostat 2022

In general, significant differences are found between North-Western Europe and the other regions, with internet access and digital skills being significantly higher in the former. When analysing by age, level of education, sex, urban status, employment status, and income level, differences across countries also become clear. Younger people, with higher education, non-female, living in urban areas, are currently a student or in employment, or are employed consistently, demonstrate higher internet access and digital skills in comparison to other demographics. While previous statistics for Europe have reported high internet access (Global Kids Online, 2021; Office of National Statistics UK, 2019; International Telecommunications Union, 2020), these levels can be misleading when taking into account the intra-

and extra-group demographics of European countries. Results in terms of overall Internet access are in accordance with previous research (88% versus 89.12% (International Telecommunications Union, 2020), yet geographical differences are glaring (75-98% access rate). To note - regardless of Internet pricing being lower and they having a higher proportion of an economically active population- the development of digital skills continues to stay behind in South-Eastern Europe.

A conglomerate of factors has to align in order for high levels of digital skills to be put into place. Nevertheless, the spread of above basic digital skills reported may demonstrate that these factors work in conjunction inconsistently or insufficiently. With the 2019 Digital Competence Framework now calling for more advanced digital competencies (Joint Research Center European Commission, 2017), this turns especially alarming considering only 34.65% (12.13%) of respondents in 2019 had higher than basic skills under the 2016 classification and these skills are mostly found in specific demographic strata (young people, people with high income, employed people and students, and people living in urban areas).

In addition to the individual factors, there are also system-level factors that must be taken into consideration. As per Greenhalgh's theory on the distribution of innovation (Greenhalg et al., 2004), it is key to consider whether – at a system level – there is a requirement for and desire to innovate, whether nations have the available resources and the needed leadership to kickoff and maintain change, and whether countries have a politico-cultural climate and demographic structure that enables the application of digital technologies. This same thinking applies when looking into the application of digital technologies across demographic groups. For example, younger people, students, and urban people have a higher probability of being raised in a digitally-enabled environment (Kickbusch et al., 2021; The Lancet Digital Health, 2021; Wong et al., 2021), which is likely to contribute to a smoother assimilation of digital technologies and, in turn, lead to greater digital skills development. In tandem, the demographics that could likely benefit most from the uptake of digital technologies are likely to be the groups that have the biggest barriers to access (Honeyman et al., 2020; van Kessel et al., 2022; Sieck et al., 2021), either due to socioeconomic status, age, health status, or additional factors.

Establishing and maintaining employment is also likely to become more challenging with increasing digitisation if the digital competence of the current and potential workforce are not suitably developed (Wong et al.,

2021). At the same time, as healthcare and public health keep digitizing, access to health services may be put into jeopardy with insufficient digital competence (Honeyman et al., 2020; Sieck et al., 2021; Kickbusch et al., 2021; Risling et al., 2019). Health is likely to further deteriorate as a result of poor digital skills if access to healthcare, social support and employment become more dependent on the possession and mastery of digital competence, additionally exacerbating already existing gaps. It is hence not only paramount from an economic perspective to invest in developing the general digital literacy and capacity, but also from a public health point of view. This applies even more so when considering the significant correlation between capital stock, income, and earnings with digital competence development. As an outcome, less developed European countries may find themselves in an unfavorable stand in relation to their developed peers. These nations will have challenges catching up, while the skill-biased technological modification may deteriorate their cross-country competitiveness.

The German Healthcare System

The adoption of digital infrastructure by physicians has increased significantly. According to a recent study, more than 90 percent of general practitioners in Germany are now connected to the telematics infrastructure, the backbone of the German digital healthcare system. Above-average connection rates occur among younger physicians in private practices, psychotherapists aged 50 or under, and medium-size to large family medicine practices.

However, digitization has not yet resulted in digital data exchange between hospitals and outpatient physicians: Ninety-five percent of communication between outpatient physicians and hospitals is still paper based. The Hospital Future Act (KHZG) has infused €4.3 billion into hospital IT to remedy this situation by accelerating the digitization of German hospitals.

Health insurers are offering their insured population ever more digital services, but so far, the uptake has been limited. For example, every statutory health insurer was required to provide its customers with an electronic health record by January 1, 2021. Six months later, fewer than 0.4 percent of the insured population of the top 20 insurers had downloaded their file.

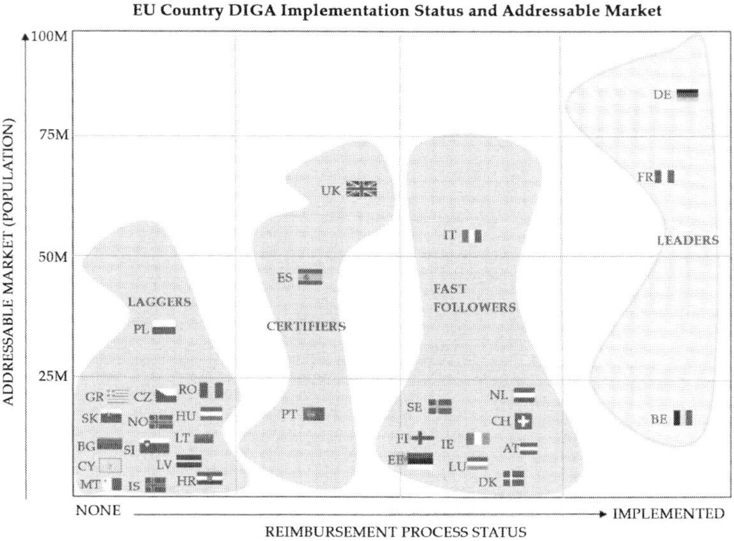

Figure 16. Reimbursement for digital health apps in the European Union.

Source: Research to Guidance, 2022

In a May 2020 survey by Doctolib, 55 percent of respondents indicated they were open to the idea of digital health offerings, but many complained of a lack of information or education about them. A study in late 2020 found that 40 percent of respondents were unaware of the forthcoming launch of downloadable electronic health records in January.

E-health apps are gaining in popularity. Between the fall of 2019 and the summer of 2021, the number of downloads of the top 40 e-health apps doubled to 2.4 million. The most popular category was online appointment booking. In the second quarter of 2021, the top five e-health apps were downloaded more than 400,000 times, a tenfold increase over the second quarter of 2019.

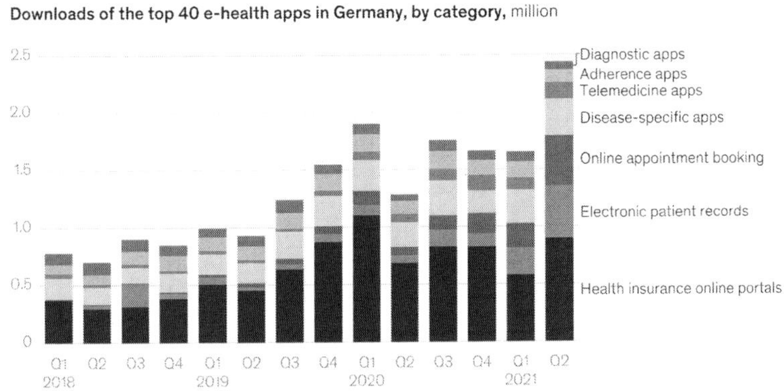

Figure 17. Digital Health Apps in Germany.

The number of German research publications about e-health solutions has increased almost sixfold in the past decade, from 20 in 2010 to 116 in 2020. This is still only half as many publications as in the United Kingdom, which has the highest number of e-health publications in Europe. Of the academic publications that assess the potential benefits of e-health, 84 percent indicate the applications have benefits, with three-quarters showing an improvement in patient outcomes. In addition, 10 percent show an improvement in cost efficiency, and 14 percent show that healthcare professionals benefit from time savings.

CURRENT SITUATION IN LOW AND MIDDLE INCOME COUNTRIES

Professionals in the health field have traditionally provided health information and training to population groups in rural areas in the Global South in the form of paper leaflets or via oral transmission. With the increased use of digital technologies, information and training may be given in innovative and more effective ways, which are likely to be more impactful on the prevention and treatment of disease.

Regardless of the significant progress achieved by some nations, various countries still need institutional backup for the creation and strengthening of country-wide digital health and/or strategic setup of digital health and the application of their action plans, which often needs greater resources and capabilities. The application of suitable digital health technologies is a main component of a country-wide strategy but can be challenging to manage particularly in low- and middle-income countries. Examining the potential of international solutions and co-services ought to be taken into account as a component of the country-wide health strategy of WHO Member States, simultaneously as creating evidence on the impact for access, cost, quality, safety and sustainability of using these international solutions in health systems within greatly diverse national contexts.

Digital health holds great potential (WHO, 2019). It may help turn health information, care, and diagnosis more accessible, for example via telemedicine (Ezell et al., 2018). This is particularly the case for people in hard-to-reach places, considering the spread of low-cost smart phones and medical tools. Digital health may allow health-care professionals and services to turn more efficient and become of higher quality. Particularly, the strengthened utilization of health information offers the potential of more tailored and coordinated attention, and improved, faster treatment at a reduced cost (Castro and Korte, 2014). AI has progressed to the point where it can handle shortages of specialists, giving reliable diagnosis and reduced-cost services in fields ranging from tuberculosis to diabetic retinopathy. Similarly, AI can use the larger availability of health information to spot and prevent emerging health concerns, including epidemics. When in combination with software, better, richer information sets permit health system managers to identify, plan, and provide resources with greater efficiency. Digital health may also speed up the medical development process (New, 2019). As an example, AI may integrate and analyze a wider range of "real-world" information from mobile and wearable technologies as well as social media, and connect it with classic lab and clinical information (Loftus, 2019).

Several of these advantages are already apparent, and hold special promise for LMICs since they can be deployed at much lower cost than traditional brick-and-mortar health services. As an indication of this, digital health technologies are nowadays undergoing a steep growth in uptake. Internationally, 44 percent of mobile users have approached a medical service provider for diagnosis or treatment by way of their mobile device (MEF, 2015). In accordance with IQVIA (a U.S. health technology firm), the amount of mHealth goods and services has doubled in the past 5 years in LMICs, with currently over 165,000 mobile applications for health services (Aiteken and Lyle, 2015). Mobile health services are more popular in LMICs, with 59 percent of users in LMICs making use of digital health apps and services, in comparison with 35 percent in high-income countries (PWC, 2012).

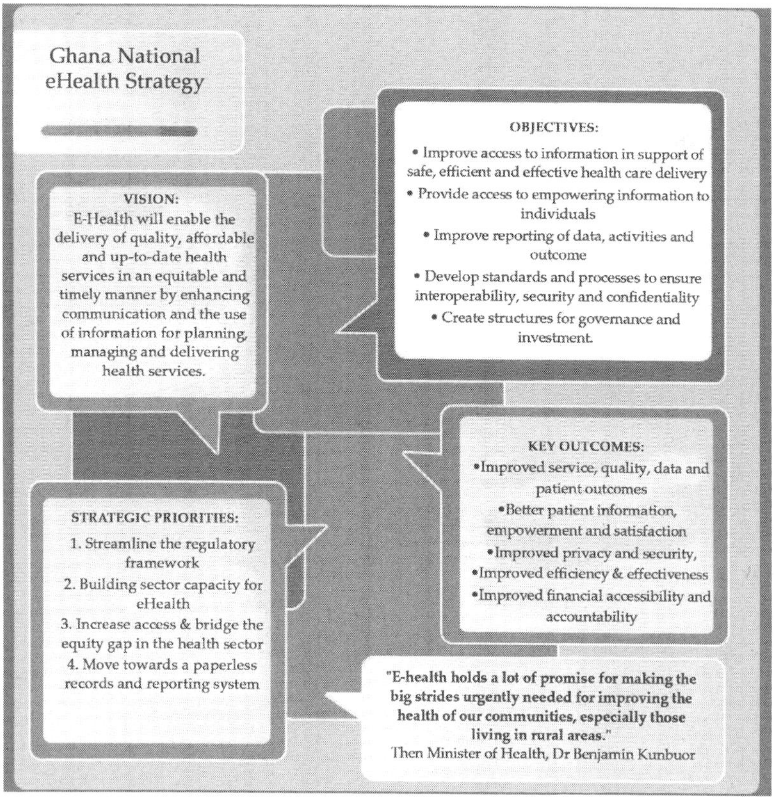

Figure 18. Ghanian National eHealth Strategy.

Source: Healthenabeled.org 2022

To carry out the potential of digital healthcare at scale, robust national partnerships and promoting environments will be needed in the majority of cases—and the effort will likely require attention on known, adaptable technologies and user-centered design. Along those critical success points, LMICs will likely be required to pay particular attention to effective capability building, sustainable business models, and detailed monitoring and evaluation.

If LMICs apply these success points, they could strengthen and widen the application of digital tools over multiple use cases in primary healthcare. LMIC governments and their partners may then keep moving toward their targets of shaping the country-wide healthcare ecosystems that link multiple healthcare journeys and aggregating information for seamless patient experiences.

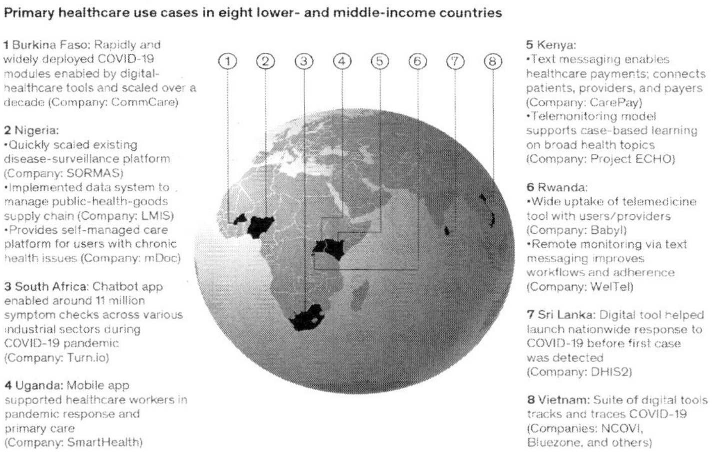

Figure 19. Primary healthcare use cases in eight lower and middle income countries.

Source: McKinsey & Company, 2022

> **Box 14. Ghana: digital skills for pharmacists**
>
> The community-based hypertension improvement project (ComHIP), in the Eastern Region of Ghana, provides capacity building to licensed medicine sellers in the community to screen for and give suitable health education and information on hypertension to their users. This program, underpinned by a comprehensive digital health platform, optimizes opportunities for screening and diagnosis of hypertension in a peri-urban area of sub-Saharan Africa, and provides closer chronic disease care to the local population. The project shows how directed training of end beneficiaries of digital health platforms may be effective in improving health outcomes.
>
> Ranking 102 of 139 in terms of networked readiness, Ghana faces a number of eHealth challenges including a shortage of skills, high ICT costs and poor infrastructure. However, uptake of mobile phones in Ghana is very high, and there is enormous potential for mHealth to help extend health information and services to the almost 50% of people living in rural areas in Ghana. A recent review of eHealth projects in Ghana found 22 separate initiatives most of which are donor funded.

DIGITAL HEALTH IN LATIN AMERICA

Addressing international health issues requires suitable utilization of available technologies. Even though digital health could strongly improve access, use, quality, and outcomes of health care, realizing this option needs a workforce which is digitally competent. There is accumulating evidence of the advantages of digital health for bettering the performance of health systems and outcomes in developed nations. Nevertheless, significant discrepancies remain in resource-constrained settings. Technological and socio-cultural disparities between different areas or between provinces within the same nation are common. Rural areas, where the promise and requirement are highest, are especially in need. In Latin America, there is a lack of training and building the capacity of digital health providers. A successful digital health ecosystem for Latin America needs culturally relevant and collaborative research and training programs in digital health. These programs must be responsive to the requirements of all relevant regional stakeholders, including government agencies, non–governmental organizations, industry, academic or research entities, professional societies, and communities.

Latin America is still seen as the most disparate region in the world (Vincens et al., 2018). According to the 2019 Global Multidimensional Poverty Index report by the United Nations Development Programme and the Oxford Poverty and Human Development Initiative, 39 million people in Latin America are living with multidimensional poverty (UNDP, 2019). Latin America is a part of the world with particular local characteristics connected to economy, employment, housing, education, cultural context, and health care (Farach et al., 2015).

Information and communication technologies may help lower those inequalities in Latin America, being key tools to promote innovation and knowledge development in societies, especially to disadvantaged groups and rural areas. Latin American countries need to properly make use of information and communication technologies to address the health needs of their peoples. In October 2019, the 57th Directing Council of the Pan American Health Organization (PAHO), through Resolution CD57/9, adopted the Plan of Action for Strengthening Information Systems for Health 2019-2023 (Farach et al., 2015) to guarantee improved collection and management of data. This was done to provide information for decision-making, policy development, monitoring, and evaluation. This highlights the need for strengthening resource capacity for the proper implementation of health information systems, considering the context, needs, vulnerabilities, and priorities of countries (Farach et al., 2015).

It has been widely accepted that health education and involvement in health promotion action will be transformed by digital innovations and that health competency increases when individuals begin utilizing digital tools to reach information and take informed decisions linked to their personal health (WHO, 2016). Nevertheless, low rates of literacy and digital competence are barriers to having access to digital information, particularly in rural sections of low-income countries (GSM, 2020). Hence, it is key that the design of a digital tool is inclusive and ascertains that beneficiaries develop the competence needed to take advantage of such digital progress (Zelezny et al., 2018).

Coming up with digital health communications for a Global South target can be difficult considering the previously mentioned gaps in literacy, digital literacy, access to internet, and access to devices. The structures of power, poverty, gender inequality, and health inequities at large, including poor infrastructure, complicate the situation for various populations, including marginalized ones. Nevertheless, the future of health education and health promotion involvement in sub-Saharan Africa may indeed be digital (Holst et al., 2020). The impact of early partnering with local decision makers and beneficiaries in a co-creation process is key for optimal results (Adam et al., 2019). In the next section, a case study from Tanzania will be discussed, followed by an illustration of how it is possible to create content for a global digital health intervention using a multi- and interdisciplinary process.

Sub-Saharan Africa is a resource-limited region that experiences a top-heavy share of the world's burden of disease. According to the World Health Organization (WHO), approximately 12% of the world's peoples live in sub-Saharan Africa, still the region suffers 27% of the world's total burden of disease (WHO, 2008). To further the situation negatively, the same region with a high burden of disease also falls behind in health information technology (HIT) which is essential in guaranteeing better patients care (Chaplin et al., 2015; Ajiboye et al., 2014; Cline and Luiz, 2013; Fraser et al., 2005; Williams and Boren, 2008; Pantuvo et al., 2011). Opportunely as well as correct patient data is key to meet the health-care requirements of any patient in any population. Medical professionals and other care providers need high quality data to make sound clinical decisions; still, their information requirements are usually not met (Williams and Boren, 2008; Simba and Mwangu 2004). This missing high quality information often makes way to reduced quality and inefficient patient management; reporting as well as clinical research is also affected negatively. The critical necessity for optimal health information systems in sub-Saharan Africa has turned into the current focus of attention.

Recently, there has been increasing interest in electronic medical records (EMRs) or electronic health records (EHR) adoption in numerous countries. This has been as a result of growing recognition that a stronger HIT is key to reaching greater quality care at reduced costs (Chaplin et al., 2015; Cline and Luiz, 2013; Fraser et al., 2005; Pantuvo et al., 2011). The International Organization for Standardization (ISO) provides a definition for an EHR as a "repository of patient data in digital form, stored and exchanged securely, and accessible by various authorized users. It contains retrospective, concurrent, and prospective information and its primary purpose is to support continuing, efficient, and quality integrated health care" (IOS, 2005).

EHR has been identified to be a key integral component of a smooth running health-care information system that assures positive health solutions (Chaplin et al., 2015; Cline and Luiz, 2013; Fraser et al., 2005; Williams and Boren 2008).

Broad research undertaken in varying health-care areas have reported that EHRs will help health professionals to minimize medical mistakes, achieve more effective care coordination, increase safety and quality, and in addition, it can lower health-care costs (Chaplin et al., 2015; Cline and Luiz, 2013; Williams and Boren, 2008; Pantuvo et al., 2011; Blaya et al., 2010; Castelnuovo et al., 2012). Health-care systems, like other industries, are data-dence organizations (Shortliffe et al., 2014). Health-care professionals require suitable information in addition to data management solutions to make optimal decisions, both while in patient care and management of the health-care system, and to communicate and track patient care processes (Shortliffe et al., 2014).

Currently, the application of an EHR includes clinical care application/functions, clinical research options, and administrative sections. The Institute of Medicine pinpoints that a more immediate access to computer-based clinical data, including laboratory and radiology outcomes, may lower redundancy and increase quality (Institute of Medicine, 2013). Likewise, the availability of complete patient health data at the point of care delivery, in combination with clinical decision support systems including those for drug prescription entry may prevent several medical errors and negative events (injuries resulting from medical management as opposed to from the original disease or condition of the patient) from taking place (Institute of Medicine, 2013; Oluoch et al., 2012).

Additionally, through a secure EHR, patient health data can be distributed among all authorized benefitialries in the health-care settings.

Computer-based reminder systems for beneficiaries and professionals may improve compliance with preventive service actions. A more advanced EHR is also paramount for various forms of biomedical and health systems research, in addition to educating users and citizens regarding health (Institute of Medicine, 2013). In addition, research undertaken by Hillestad *et al.* on the probable health outcomes and cost reducing benefit of EHR implementation revealed that broad implementation of EHR would lower health-care costs by over $81 billion yearly in the United States (Hillestad et al., 2005). Generally, the significance of EHR in increasing user safety and quality care, minimizing medical mistakes and health-care costs should not be overstressed so also the benefits of its broad utilization in sub-Saharan Africa.

Numerous industrialized countries including Canada, the United Kingdom, and the United States of America have either adopted or are in the process of adopting an EHR system due to its possible benefits (Williams and Boren, 2008; Pantuvo et al., 2011; Williams and Boren, 2008). Nevertheless, there is a maximum level of adoption of EHR in sub-Saharan African nations, regardless of the numerous benefits deriving from its adoption. The research carried out by Akanbi *et al.* on the utilization of EHR in sub-Saharan Africa demonstrated that the adoption of EHRs in sub-Saharan Africa is mostly driven by HIV management international programs such as President's Emergency Plan for AIDS Relief HIV program (Akanbi et al., 2012). Application is still, nevertheless, laging (Fraser et al., 2005; Pantuvo et al., 2011; Akanbi et al., 2012). Further, many of the most commonly available electronic functionalities with EHR in this part of the world are more administrative, rather than medical (Akanbi et al., 2012).

The components that stop the adoption of EHR in different health-care areas in Africa have not been amply researched. Pinpointing factors that have an impact on EHR adoption in this region of the world is key to inform all health stakeholders, policy makers, researchers, and academic health organizations that train medical staff, pharmacists, nurses, and laboratory scientists, to mention but a few. To answer the query as to why low utilization of EHR in this region, it is important to highlight and comprehend the components that limit wide adoption of EHR. Further, to speed up wider adoption of EHR, there is a requirement to have a better grasp of the EHR adoption facilitating components.

Case study: the Tanzanian Healthcare System

About 70% of the Tanzanian peoples live in rural areas and mostly depend on primary health facilities to cover their health necessities. The principal health facilities in Tanzania are categorized into dispensaries and health centers. Dispensaries facilitate a basic plethora of preventive, health promotion, curative and maternal and child health (MCH) care, while health centers in turn provide inpatient and a higher level of delivery care and are staffed by a greater variety of higher qualified health professional between 39 up to 52 compared to the dispensaries which have between 15 up to 20 health service employees. District hospitals function as a referral for primary health care (Kapologwe et al, 2020).

Popular programs that have been utilized in Tanzania to relieve pressure on the professionally trained healthcare providers include the adoption of community health workers (CHWs) and other close-to-community (CTC) health facilitators. CTC provider programmes have facilitated strong gains, such as those focused on child health—lowering malnutrition and neonatal and under-five mortality and giving community case handling of childhood health conditions. Gains have also been seen in lowering maternal mortality and optimizing access to family planning services, spreading the use of insecticide-treated bed nets for malaria control, and promoting testing and delivering cost- effective, community-based management of tuberculosis (Datiko et al., 2020). For HIV prevention and care, CTC facilitators have been reported to be effective in improving HIV-related knowledge (Marcos et al., 2012), lessening risky sexual behaviors, augmenting antiretroviral treatment (ART) utilization (Sarna et al., 2013), providing home- based care, and optimizing access and quality of care (Cellatti et al., 2010).

Nevertheless, CTC programmes have many obstacles. The official status, reach of training, and compensation for CTC providers are wide ranging, depending on whether they are officially employed by the government, acting as volunteers, or are involved through non-governmental organizations (NGOs). Remuneration can range from modest salaries (Hermann et al., 2009; Robinson et al., 1990) to performance-based incentives (Alam et al., 2014; Gopalan et al., 2012), community contributions (Haile et al., 2014), or incentives including t- shirts or bicycles or non-material recognition (Brunie et al., 2014; Perez et al., 2009). Several, low- and middle-income governments have difficulties paying salaried community workers and do not have the setup to absorb and pay or otherwise create incentives for volunteers (Bhutta et al., 2010). The productivity, motivation, and long-term success of CTC providers may vary and be affected by their level of remuneration or incentives given.

CTC providers also encounter difficulties from their communities; they can at times not be accepted, recognized, or supported by their serving communities if their selection is done without considering socio-cultural contexts. As an example, in Afghanistan, the involvement of a woman CHW was reported to facilitate adoption of modern family planning methods, antenatal care, and skilled birth processes, while the involvement of a male CHW did not have the same effect possibly because of the socio-cultural norms that determine how men and women interact (Viswananthan et al., 2011). Community participation in the work of CTC providers may have a beneficial effect. Similar acceptance/rejection of digitally-facilitated health care can arise if socio-cultural considerations of targeted communities are not present.

In Tanzania, community health employees and health institutions, as well as nongovernmental organizations, have usually given health promotion and education verbally or in printed form (leaflets, billboards, banners, posters, etc) to communities and populations (HSSP 2020). The Tanzanian digital landscape is quickly changing, and in tandem with noteworthy economic development (WB, 2022), an increase in adoption of mobile phones in both urban and rural regions and one of the most wide-reaching mobile markets in sub-Saharan Africa has been appreciated (GSM Association, 2019). Tanzania, East Africa's third largest economy with 54.2 million people, had 43.6 million mobile phone subscribers in June 2018 (approximately 80% of the population), in comparison to 40.1 million a year earlier and in contrast to just 10.2 out of 40.7 million people (25% of the population) in 2007 (National Bureau of Statistics Tanzania, 2021). Nevertheless, only 13% of subscribers reported to have a smartphone in 2017 (Pew Research Center, 2018). The Tanzania Digital Health Strategy 2019-2024 aims to increase the use of digital health technologies to champion healthy behavior via access to health information, education, and communication (Ministry of Health, Community Development, Gender, Elderly and Children, 2019).

The Tanzanian government plans to scale up and strengthen the achievements of the past eHealth Strategy 2013-2018, which set up diverse electronic data systems (such as the use of television, radio, social media, etc) to give and encourage health education. Even though community-based health services target health promotion and disease prevention, mobile health and social media are able to be used more widely to bring quality health education, information, and communication, empowering people to adopt healthier ways of life and to develop their health literacy. Health communications with an impact are clearly required in the international fight against infectious diseases such as HIV/AIDS, tuberculosis (TB), and zoonosis (diseases that affect animals and humans) including Taenia solium cysticercosis and taeniasis (TSCT) and anthrax. The Tanzanian Health Sector Strategic Plan states that the disease prevention strategy for HIV/AIDS and TB have been carried out successfully in the regions of early detection and treatment. Nevertheless, additional improvements are required in the area of prevention (Ministry of Health and Social Welfare. 2015). As for TSCT, which is highlighted as a neglected tropical condition by the WHO (2021), prevention is paramount since the disease is highly endemic in Tanzania (Ngowi et al., 2019). Anthrax is an ongoing neglected zoonotic condition, endemic in the African zone and current in the north of Tanzania (especially in the Maasai communities) where regular outbreaks in livestock, wildlife, and humans have made clear the need to fortify prevention strategies (Mwakapege 2018).

The Non-discriminating access for Digital Inclusion (DigI) program, in which the creation of health communications represents a typical multi- and interdisciplinary program funded as an innovation project, with the objective of linking rural villages to digital information. The DigI project's multi- and interdisciplinary composition, including 11 partners from 8 countries, covers scientists in the areas of humanities, social sciences, formal sciences, and applied sciences. These key areas cover a variety of sub-areas: medicine and health, epidemiology, public health, veterinary medicine, electronic engineering, visual and creative arts with graphic and interaction design, human-computer interaction, communication, education or educational technology, information science, internet science, and ethics. Input from anthropology, human geography, health psychology, and sociology of health and illness have been used in the various steps of planning and implementation of this project. Through a collaboration of Tanzanian, German, Norwegian, Rwandan, and American participants, the aim is to develop digital health communications by converting printed flyers into digital form including animated videos (animations), quizzes, graphics, and texts.

Most of the DigI participants either are part of the information technology (IT) and design task force, or the health task force. The Tanzanian and

German program collaborators with training in health and medicine bring expertise on HIV/AIDS, TB, TSCT, and anthrax. The participants were able to rely on their many years of experience working with each condition in the target communities. The prioritized conditions in the DigI project are endemic in the selected geographical regions and hence are key conditions in the Tanzanian public health setting. All these conditions are of high priority and need preventive strategies such as information dissemination to various population groups.

A digital health education tool, the DigI platform (Digi, 2021), was devised and created from 2017 to 2019 by the DigI workforce. It is made up of a dashboard where users are able to move through numerous pages with facts about the condition. The tool features texts, quizzes, graphics, and animated videos that are accessible for everyone. The tool with the health communications was set up as part of an information spot (InfoSpot) in the rural villages of Selela and Esilalei in the Arusha areas (for anthrax) and Migoli and Izazi in the Iringa areas (for HIV/AIDS, TB, and TSCT) in November 2019. It is possible to access the health information on the platform, even if the beneficiary is not linked to the internet, since the platform is also locally stored on a village server.

Development of the Digital Content in Tanzania

In the context of the data in the print materials, the digitization process in Tanzania began by the development of a non-complicated story communicating the key health teachings, with components of storytelling to keep the *users'* attention. *Users* is the term given to "members of the public that are potential or current users of health services, including promotion activities". The stories were inspired by a rural Tanzanian village-life setting, turning them into plausible and realistic for the users, with a focus on maintaining the story's simplicity, honesty, and emotional value. In the context of these made-up stories, storyboards (drawings with captions below each image or scene) were developed to illustrate the narrative so the DigI team could give more informed feedback. Following the approval of the storyboards, the second step is to develop animated videos with voiceover narrations in both English and Swahili. The DigI team iterated a series of design-test-evaluate-design cycles, whereby a story was tested and improved accordingly. The digitization process is illustrated in Figure X below.

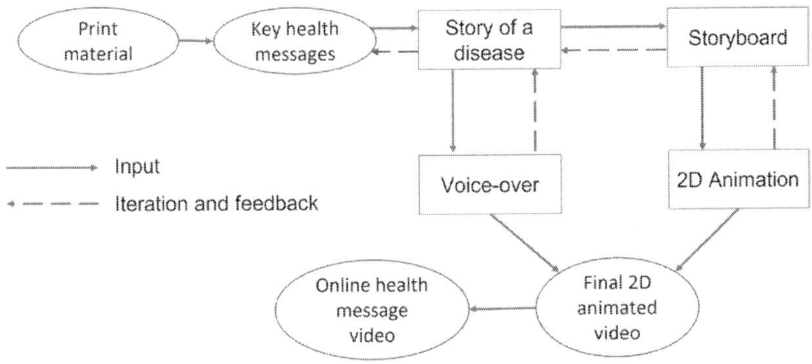

Figure 20. Health message digitization process.

Source: healthcatalyst.com

The specific approach to content development was set up based on the internal debate. The objective was to meet users' needs, values, language, and culture and highlighted the rural Tanzanian setting all through the development steps. In the following 10 sections, each phase of the methodological approach is described in detail, with general advice and takeaway messages for each section.

A Local Needs Assessment

A human-centered design method (ISo 2019) is needed when creating apps to cover individual requirements. In some projects, surveys are carried out at the start to collect clients' requirements in the project locations, and a participatory and community-led approach is deliberately selected over the introduction of an external digital health program (Cornwall and Jewkers, 1995). Prior to the development of the digital health communications, various location visits are to be undertaken by health- and IT-researchers in the program. Throughout these visits, local requirements and preferences are collected via discussions with community stakeholders, including village leaders, health workers, and other members of the community. During the requirements evaluation, it became clear to the DigI workforce that the most suitable health education format was animation. The locals voiced the challenges with low literacy in rural societies, suggesting cartoons or films for teaching about health. Tanzanian Swahili was clearly a must, as the great majority of people in Tanzania do not speak English. Even though some ethnic groups have their own languages, the majority of people understand Tanzanian Swahili. Some village stakeholders also voiced the requirement for additional information, including village news, village meetings, and agriculture information.

The overall advice based on previous experience is to devote plenty of time to exploring the local requirements and involving local stakeholders as participants to develop the process and tailor the end product from the very beginning.

Identification of Government-Approved Health Promotion Materials in a Non Digital Format

Health strategies and regulations may vary from one nation to another, and it is key to pay attention to the progress that has already been made by policy makers, health workers, and researchers at a country level when mapping the local environment. Newly developed video animations represent up-to-date, high-quality, and straight forward health communications that are developed in the context of approved health information materials, as a point of start for digitization. The information is modified from leaflets, posters, brochures, banners, guidelines, and strategies, all succinctly reviewed for key health communications targeting the public health audience. Messages from the Ministry of Health, Community Development, Gender, Elderly and Children–approved health education for HIV and TB were used. HIV health education communications were obtained from the National AIDS Control Programme (Ministry of Health, Community Development, Gender, Elderly and Children 2017). Additionally, posters and presentations were collected from the National Tuberculosis and Leprosy Control Programme, whereas the National Strategic Plan V (2015-2020) for Tuberculosis and Leprosy (The United Republic of Tanzania. Ministry of Health and Social Welfare 2015). This information has been used for the development of various documentaries. The health educational material for TSCT was provided by the Cysticercosis Working Group in Eastern and Southern Africa, and the United Republic of Tanzania One Health Strategic Plan 2015-2020 (One Health Strategic Plan 2015) was considered for inspiration. The handouts for the prevention and control of anthrax in humans and animals were collectively prepared by the Ministry of Health, Community Development, Gender, Elderly and Children, Ministry of Livestock and Fisheries, and the Ministry of Natural Resources and Tourism supported by the Food and Agriculture Organization of the United Nations and WHO country offices in Tanzania, applying a One Health approach. The hard copies were turned into soft copies and distributed to the DigI team to turn them into digital formats.

From this point on, it is generally suggested that care be taken and respect kept toward the national health authorities. National guidelines, programs and regulations may contain important health communications to be conveyed, particularly to target populations, due to context-specific reasons, and may vary from international and global guidelines.

Identification of Key Health Messages

The next step is to establish the most important information that it is desired to convey, depending on the health area and aimed demographic. For example, it might be desired to address infectious diseases for a rural population in Tanzania, hence pushing the key health communications into the following categories:

(1) frequency of the disease
(2) origin or transmission of the disease
(3) signs or symptomatology of the disease
(4) management of the disease
(5) prevention

Once the categories are prioritized, the main health messages should be extracted from the materials described in the previous section. During this process, short paragraphs, highlighting the key messages for each domain, should be developed. This is transferable across all health areas: it is important to keep it short and simple.

The starting category aims to increase regional awareness and covers health messages about the disease and its prevalence in the region. The second category has information on how diseases spread and infect others. The third category describes the signs and symptoms of the disease, to help with timely detection and handling of the disease. Health communications encourage and create motivation for users to look for medical advice if symptoms are present. The fourth category is linked to the treatment of diseases. The final and likely most influential domain covers information on how individuals can achieve protection for themselves and their communities and how the disease can be stopped from spreading across individuals and within population groups.

The overall advice from previous experience is to rather focus exclusively on only the key messages at once and maintain the communication short and simple so as to avoid overloading the beneficiaries with information.

Development of a Practical and Engaging Story, Easy to Understand for the Public

Historically, humans have acquired knowledge from stories. Stories can be an impactful way to transmit information and specific communications to other people (Schank et al., 2002). Storytelling techniques can effectively be used to develop a relatable everyday narrative story that users are able to recognize and relate to. In the case of the illustrations below, all animations were developed by the DigI team; nevertheless, some project-specific partners led the process of developing the story. The first run was discussed by the DigI taskforce. From there, health content was reviewed by the health task force. Following a draft of the content of the story, a second team labored on developing a document that included the script for each story. Each script was made up of facts regarding the health condition and a creative mix of characters, actions, and location settings within the situation of a village in rural Tanzania. The scripts were closely revised by Tanzanian DigI members to check for local compatibility.

> This is the story of how tapeworms affected my village.
> My grandpa had been feeling poorly for a few weeks. He had terrible headaches, blurred vision and confusion. Then grandpa had seizures. I brought him to the dispensary right away. After checking him and running some tests, the doctor told us his symptoms were caused by tapeworms. She said, my grandpa must have eaten or drunken the tiny tapeworm eggs without realizing it and gotten sick. The larvae settled in my grandpa's brain causing seizures, bad headaches and confusion. They even settled in his eyes causing blurred vision and he could go blind if not treated. (Excerpt from the script from "The Story of Tapeworms")

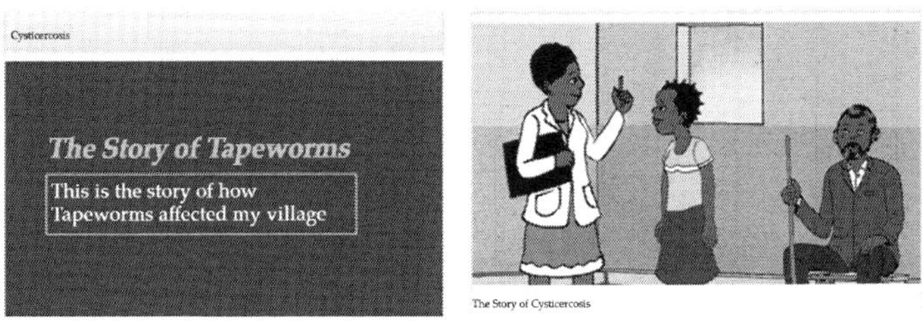

Figure 21. Excerpt from "The Story of Tapeworms".

Source: Holst et al., 2021

The stories should generally be presented by a narrator and make references to members of a family in addition to the community facing the addressed health condition. The narrative covers elements to attract and keep users' attention by providing a description of routine activities and the realities of life in a rural sub-Saharan setting.

The overall recommendations based on previous experience from story creation is to invite a range of stakeholders to review the scripts. Experts and community members can contribute in equal amounts, but with diverse perspectives. Experts must guarantee that the health information is being presented in a suitable manner and that no key information is left out, whereas community members may identify words and phrases that are hard to understand. It may be of use to ask questions such as "Are all key messages promoted clearly? Is the language understandable and the story credible?"

Drafting of a Storyboard for an Animated Video with Review, Feedback, and Revisions

Following the script's approval, a storyboard must be developed if the objective is to generate a film or animation. A storyboard is composed of a drawing containing text below, illustrating scenes (i.e. farming scenes) that are feasibly common in rural settings. It is advisable to distribute the storyboards with the aimed demographics at an early stage so as to have some feedback at this stage of the design process. For example, in one project the plan was to use simplified human line drawings, yet following the feedback session it was advised by the local population to include more genuine characters to promote greater involvement from the communities when viewing the animations. Additional feedback from the same group included a suggestion to make the characters and environment closer in similarity to those found in rural Tanzania. This included, for example, modifying the façade of the health facilities and the attire of the characters. The main health messages from the written material were not altered, as these messages were approved, and modifying them would require new ethical approval. Following the process of design-test-evaluate-design, an animated video can be created based on the original script, revisions, and feedback from expert team members and local community members.

The overall advice based on previous experience is to establish the storyboards as soon as the script has been approved. The storyboards allow for the animation visualization to be more realistic and can be effective in highlighting scenes of importance for important message uptake. It is of benefit to include target users at this time to achieve recognizability and authenticity in different scenes.

Forward and Backward Translation

Working in two languages may present a challenge and can make the process more complex. Thus, professional translators with experience in the field are required to ascertain that translation is uniformed throughout the diverse versions of the script. In the example of the programs in Tanzania, health communications and story scripts were developed in English followed by a translation to Swahili for the desired population. The process went like this:

- English health messages and story scripts were given to a person to translate them into Swahili.
- Thereafter, the Swahili versions were given to another person to translate them back into English.
- Further, the back translation was compared with the original English health messages and story scripts to ensure that the messages were the same.
- The Swahili messages were also read by the medical doctors who spoke Swahili to ensure that the messages had the same information as the English messages.

It has been previously reported that modifications of the script are usually carried out numerous times, including following translation; hence, it is important to ascertain that the final script represents the same key messages in all languages involved.

Audio Recording of the Story in Both Languages

Once the script and translations are completed, it is time to record the story. Even though it is suggested that a professional recording studio be employed, the key factor is to be able to record the audio file free from background noise and with a clear and understandable narrator. Technically, recording itself is a straightforward process. It should be emphasized that the narrators must speak slowly and clearly in an informal tone. The audio file should be carefully revised by team members who are native or near-natives speakers of the languages involved. It is recommended that particular attention be paid to the initial revision process of the audio file. There are cases where a written sentence conveys health messages more effectively than when reading aloud, and to save costs, it may be useful to read the script aloud to team members prior to recording it.

Finalization and Presentation of the Animation

After the voice recordings and animation scenes are final, the animated video can be fully produced and disseminated with the team for revision and improvement. After at least 2 rounds of revisions, the final animated videos can be produced and then presented to an audience, in this case in rural Tanzania. In Tanzania, the example, The *Story of Tapeworms* animation was completed in 2018. The *Story of HIV/AIDS* animation and the *Story of TB*animation were finalized in March 2019. The *Story of Anthrax* animation was completed in May 2019. Generally, this phase can be expensive, but it is worthwhile to address small difficulties in the final product, which can be of importance for health information transfer.

Development of Relevant Questions Related to the Health Messages in Each Domain

To promote knowledge acquisition, it can be useful to come up with questions from digital health messages, including animations, and present them to the audience in the form of a quiz, for example, following the audience view of the animation. Knowledge questions related to different diseases from the key health messages for each domain can be derived. These questions should be constructed for research purposes to evaluate user's knowledge prior to and following the exposure to the digital health messages in a quantitative study. The same questions can be published on the platform in a quiz format so that users are able to test their own learning. It is important to ensure that the questions do not use medically advanced wording or information. Specifically, the health task force should evaluate their quality as they relate to the health content, and the social scientists should make the questions easier to understand for the clients.

The experience is that the questions created should not be too difficult, but should reflect the health messages, and work as reinforcers of the information provided in the animations.

Development of Web and Mobile Apps to Access the Digital Health Messages

In the Global South, lacking information may be a bottleneck in the prevention of diseases. Animations and other digital forms for health education in the regional language are only useful if they are available for the target audience. Thus, in the DigI project, it was just as important to create an easy-to-use digital platform so that community members in rural zones could access health information. Key requisites for the platform to be successful included that it would be simple to learn *how to use* it and that it could be utilized with a minimal level of digital literacy. Since the majority of people are likely to access health messages on a mobile phone, the *mobile-first design* approach is recommended, with the development of a responsive web application and an Android-based mobile app. The web application displays health messages in an interactive way, whereby a user is shown an animated video, key health messages, graphics, and a quiz.

As part of the human-centered design process (ISO, 2019), the project workforce specified the needs of web and mobile app systems based on feedback from village stakeholders in Migoli and Izazi in the Iringa area. The proposed designs were iteratively improved from a conceptual design to low-fidelity prototypes and high-fidelity interactive prototypes using Adobe XD (Adobe Xd, 2021). The low-fidelity prototypes were uncomplicated sketches and wireframes to illustrate early user interface designs for discussions in the DigI team. These assisted in gathering user input and suggestions on what could be better. In addition, high-fidelity prototypes presented more enriched user interfaces, with interactivity for the test users to experience the interaction with the designed tool. In addition to testing and assessing by the medical workforce and additional team members in Tanzania, user-based testing was carried out using the IT task force to discover potential usability problems. User testing targets efficiency, effectiveness, and overall user satisfaction. Using purposive sampling, a total of 12 test users, aged 15-25 years, participated in 2 rounds of usability testing conducted in Kigali (Rwanda) as part of an iterative design procedure. All assessment users had an education level of post primary school, but none had completed secondary school. The first high-fidelity prototypes were assessed by 8 participants (3 women and 5 men) in October 2018, and the second improved versions of the web and mobile app were assessed by 4 participants in July 2019. The findings showed that it was easy to access health information on the platform, view the videos, and read key health messages for different health conditions. Test users reported that it was uncomplicated to navigate the system and that the content was set up in a logical manner. Nevertheless, part of the respondents mentioned that "it was hard to find the videos" in the initial versions of the platform. Thus, global navigation was redesigned, adding a direct link to a page with videos for all health conditions at the top menu. Test users additionally proposed making two separate videos for each health condition: one video for a story and another with only the health messages. Nevertheless, after discussions, the project taskforce decided to keep 1 integrated animation per health condition, not too long to maintain the audience's attention. Additionally, test participants suggested extra requirements, including the possibility of self-assessment through search functionality on symptoms. This indicated the participant's perception of the platform as a health system. Subsequently, design constraints were employed to stop users from attempting to do anything that the system is not designed for, to make clear that the aim of the platform is to facilitate health information as opposed to providing a medical diagnosis. It is in this regard that global navigation includes links to *Health Information*, covering videos, text, and quizzes, as well as a contact form, without a search bar. Still, given the limited screen size of mobile devices, the mobile app has a search field to help users easily find information on the health conditions included in the platform.

The test volunteers were allocated a number of tasks to carry out, while a usability assessor observed their performance to identify any errors with the software under testing. Although posttest focus group discussions were carried out to gain insights into users' impressions, a self-reporting web-based questionnaire helped to compile users' opinions on a Likert scale. The resulting web designs have been deployed on village servers so that users can access health messages (Digi, 2021) from an InfoSpot free of charge, or on the internet. The user can explore video animations, key health information, and quizzes when clicking on the different health conditions. The cholera animation was developed by The Global Health Media Project prior to the DigI project and was added on the platform as an extra. The dashboard additionally gives the user an option to watch more videos.

Since an increasing number of individuals have access to low-cost mobile devices, an Android mobile app was also developed to show the same health messages as on the platform. Mobile app users have the option to download all the videos on their devices so that they can view them without an internet connection or being close to the InfoSpot. One of the possible contexts for using the app is that someone visits an InfoSpot with Wi-Fi, then downloads the app and downloads all videos for viewing at a later time together with the family back home.

Based on the experience, it is recommended for digital health content developers to evaluate the access and context that beneficiaries have to any digital information source. Digital health education programs are only useful if the target demographic group is able to access health messages either supervised or unsupervised.

GOVERNANCE AND WORKFORCE

Governance and Workforce is the strategic leadership and oversight of digital health systems that guarantees the policy and regulatory environment of health systems protects privacy, security, stewardship and accountability. Governance places priority on a sustainable, high-performing team that is ready to deliver digitally-enabled health services. The future of sustainable, high- performing digital health ecosystems needs unique governance setups to revolutionize workplace environments. These digitally-enabled environments, in turn, allow for care delivery models that are data-driven, and guided by robust data stewardship, policy and decision-making processes.

Governance and Workforce are measured by the following:

Stewardship refers to the leadership, culture, vision and objectives necessary to support digital health. It covers the accountability frameworks and management procedures including the responsibility of planning, building, running, and monitoring digital health in addition to the resources and expertise to assess and use new technologies. The adoption of new digital tools is based on evidence and best practices to back up a system-wide adoption and scalable utilization. Criteria in alignment with the utilization of information and digital technologies are guided by, and inform, best-practice decision-making to optimize quality of care.

Policy and decision-making describe the assessment, learning and feedback, resource allocation, and coordination employed for governance processes that cover policy and decision-making necessary to support digital health transformation. Policy and decision-making procedures include evidence-based digital health strategy, alignment of digital processes, value-based health system incentives and frameworks targeting outcomes. The impact of digital transformation needs policy frameworks that support and incentivize performance (e.g. efficiency, productivity, quality and cost) outcomes, and allow health system stakeholders to develop and maintain meaningful relationships with the people and populations health systems serve.

Transparency supports connectivity and relationships with individuals and communities, including digitally-enabled communication and transparency of quality, safety, and performance outcomes. Each individual is considered a partner in healthcare whereby governance and oversight guarantees transparent access to personal health data and health system level performance results, in addition to equality in access to healthcare services, data, and digitally-enabled care provision.

Workforce capacity and competency is the quick evolution of digital health ecosystems that requires knowledge, skills and abilities across the workforce to support and enable adoption of digital health strategies to support person-enabled care focused on health and wellness. Workforce policies support and retain a high-performing workforce that is incentivized to design, take up and scale digitally-enabled care processes and operational strategies focused on outcomes, value and impact for people, populations and operational performance that advances health system sustainability.

DIGITAL HEALTH COMPETENCY FRAMEWORK

Internationally, healthcare firms value how eHealth may be able to allow them to transform the care process and optimize results. In the economic climate experienced today, it is paramount that eHealth resources are aimed at those areas which will deliver top benefits to users, improving safety and efficiency of the delivery of service. The importance of the role of clinicians in this process is now increasingly recognised.

4Establishing a digitally-ready workforce is turning into a key priority for addressing the difficult challenges in health care worldwide (Gray et al., 2016). Modern health care currently incorporates a vast amount of eHealth technologies that can be used for:

(1) monitoring, tracking, and informing health;

(2) interacting for health including using digital technologies to allow health communication among practitioners and across health professionals and users or patients;

(3) data that allows health via collecting, managing, and using health information to improve outcomes (Shaw et all., 2017).

Digital health has been identified as impactful in recent health reforms, with the potential to allow for more efficient, cost-effective care with better outcomes (Li et al., 2017; Jolly, 2011). In that way, health services now expect health professionals, new graduates, and experienced workforce alike, to be eHealth competent within practice across diverse digital health environments (Li et al., 2017).

With the digitization of healthcare and the ample availability of Web-based applications, a broad collection of skills is key to properly use said facilities.

The health, activity, and participation issues highlighted within the literature regarding digital health include the following 6 categories:

- health information management,
- communication,
- professionalism,
- information systems and technologies,
- patient focus
- health analytics

These categories are described in the Table below.

Table 2. Categorization of core domains of digital health competencies

Category	Summary	References
Health information management	Recording and storing health information in electronic systems, data quality, and information governance	Gray et al., 2014 Archer et al., 2011 Barakat et al., 2013 Britt eta l., 2016 Cannoly et al., 2008 Crawford et al., 2016 Gilstand et al., 2014 Gray et al., 2015 Honey et al., 2017 Klecum et al., 2014 Procter 2017 Röhrig et al., 2013 van Houwelingen et al., 2016 Värri et al., 2016
Communication	Using digital technologies to support interprofessional relationships, consumer-provider relationships, and multi-professional care coordination	Gray et al., 2014 Archer et al., 2011 Barakat et al., 2013 Britt eta l., 2016 Cannoly et al., 2008 Crawford et al., 2016 Gilstand et al., 2014 Gray et al., 2015 Honey et al., 2017 Klecum et al., 2014 Procter 2017 Röhrig et al., 2013 van Houwelingen et al., 2016 Värri et al., 2016

Professionalism	Critical appraisal, evidence-based practice, eHealth literacy, continued professional development, ethical use of information, and management and leadership	Gray et al., 2014 Archer et al., 2011 Barakat et al., 2013 Britt eta l., 2016 Cannoly et al., 2008 Crawford et al., 2016 Gilstand et al., 2014 Gray et al., 2015 Honey et al., 2017 Klecum et al., 2014 Röhrig et al., 2013 van Houwelingen et al., 2016 Värri et al., 2016 Friedman et al., 2016 Jogerst et al., 2015 Biggins et al., 2017 Susskind et al., 2018
Information systems and technology	Using information systems and technologies to support routine clinical care, business processes, and patient-centered service provision	Gray et al., 2014 Archer et al., 2011 Barakat et al., 2013 Britt eta l., 2016 Cannoly et al., 2008 Gilstand et al., 2014 Honey et al., 2017 Klecum et al., 2014 Röhrig et al., 2013 van Houwelingen et al., 2016 Värri et al., 2016 Friedman et al., 2016 Jogerst et al., 2015 Susskind et al., 2018
Patient focus	Patient empowerment, use of technology for self-management and wellness, patient eHealth literacy, and education	Gray et al., 2014 Archer et al., 2011 Barakat et al., 2013 Britt eta l., 2016 Cannoly et al., 2008 Gilstand et al., 2014 Honey et al., 2017 Klecum et al., 2014 Röhrig et al., 2013 van Houwelingen et al., 2016 Värri et al., 2016 Friedman et al., 2016 Jogerst et al., 2015 Susskind et al., 2018

Health analytics	Use of data analytics in practice for informed decision making, quality improvement, service planning, and delivery	Gray et al., 2014 Archer et al., 2011 Barakat et al., 2013 Britt eta l., 2016 Cannoly et al., 2008 Gilstand et al., 2014 Honey et al., 2017 Klecum et al., 2014 Röhrig et al., 2013 van Houwelingen et al., 2016 Värri et al., 2016 Friedman et al., 2016 Jogerst et al., 2015 Susskind et al., 2018

Existing Digital Health Competency Frameworks

United Kingdom

A digital competency framework for Allied Health Professionals was published byHealth Education England, developed as part of the Topol Digital Health Fellowship programme.

With 223,991 Allied Health Professionals (AHP) in their registry, the framework has been created to provide support for the fortification of digital competence; the knowledge and skills connected with digital technology in practice.

Created over a year, via numerous rounds of analysis and development, a compilation of 124 competencies across 10 domains were prioritized. The competencies are grouped as being 'compulsory', 'voluntary' or 'un-required' for the AHP role.

The 10 digital competency competencies are:

1. General: including attitudes, behaviors and fundamental skills
2. Information management / Clinical informatics: covering types, uses, structures, regulation and policies
3. Records evaluation and plans: electronic health record system focused, including capturing structured or unstructured information
4. Transfer of Care: the knowledge and skills needed to effectively transfer or share patient information across systems

5 Medicines management and optimisation: including the use of effective drug management systems (e.g. electronic prescription services, electronic or automated dispensing)
6. Orders and results management: including digital tools which allow for the requesting, reporting or reviewing the results of medical testing
7. Assets and resource optimisation: business-related and personal competencies
8. Decision support: targeting the use of systems which advise clinical reasoning and decision making in practice via the incorporation of evidence based guidelines and recommendations
9. Digital therapeutics: a broad collection of digital tools integrated into clinical practices in support of normal therapy and care
10. Meta-competencies: the knowledge and skills including leadership and behavioral characteristics which are needed to facilitate organizational or departmental digital transformation.

The framework was developed by Christopher Tack, clinical specialist physiotherapist and digital leader for Allied Health Professionals at Guy's and St Thomas' NHS FT, work carried out as part of the Topol Digital Health Fellowship, on behalf of Health Education England and NHS England.

The digital competency areas have the objective of supporting AHPs including Art Therapists, Dieticians, Drama Therapists, Occupational Therapists, Operating Department Practitioners Orthoptists, Orthotists/ Prosthetists Osteopaths, Music Therapists Paramedics, Physiotherapists, Podiatrists/ Chiropodists Radiographers (Diagnostic & Therapeutic) and Speech and Language Therapists.

Allied Health Professions (AHP) Digital competency framework (Graphic)

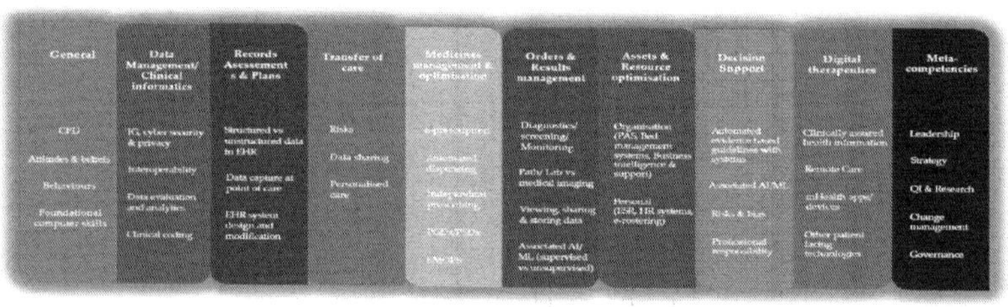

Figure 22. The Allied Health Professions Framework.

Source: Allied Health Professions, 2022

Developing the digital competency framework in the UK

A group of 40 allied health professions was gathered, covering all of the AHP areas. The expert group carried out a three round Delphi investigation to create, ratify and specify the competencies linked with their professional areas.

Round one was made up of reviews of a preliminary list of competencies separated into 93 competencies across 10 areas. The preliminary list was transferred from an analysis of the HEE digital capabilities framework and the NHS England AHP Digital Framework. Expert group members were requested to review the competencies, and make modifications and additions to the list to cover their application of digital technology in practice (specific to their professional role, or to the wider roles of AHPs).

Round two was made up of a review of the new list of 124 competencies across 11 areas and rating the applicability and relevance of each competency for each role between band 3 and band 9 (Agenda for Change pay model) specific to their profession.

Round three was made up of the ratification of the choices selected in round 2, in the context of the coronavirus pandemic, and the digital transformation changes which took place in NHS services in response to this event.

On the basis of these ongoing rounds of analysis, the AHP digital competency framework was created, covering 124 competencies within 10 domains. This document describes the whole of the framework. Nevertheless, for each banding between 3 and 9, the framework has also been altered to identify to which profession and banding each competency is compulsory, voluntary or unrequired. This will permit the implementation of the framework into the Health Education England (HEE) self-assessment tool for digital literacy, and for each profession/ band to be assessed at the appropriate level. The HEE tool can then direct users to specific learning dependent upon the summary of their self-assessment across the framework domains.

United States

USAID and digital health

Addressing the health challenges of the 21st Century necessitates pulling together the full potential of technological modifications to put aside old scourges and newer threats to public health alike. In regions where the U.S. Agency for International Development (USAID) works, digital technologies–including mobile phones, Internet-based services, and digital data systems–are becoming even more critical components of said transformation.

When applied to health, new technologies may improve disease-surveillance, extend and expand the care delivery, support remote health professionals, and empower individuals to become informed custodians of their own health and wellness. USAID plays a key role in molding this journey forward, and aims to integrate the smart use of digital technologies into all of their health programs.

USAID is working towards developing an international setup in which advances in digital technologies are leveraged to aid people in accessing the information and services they require to live healthy and prosperous lives.

The Agency's first dedicated policy guidance for its investments in digital technologies that provide support for health programs in its partner countries has been published under the name *Accelerating the Journey to Self-Reliance Through Strategic Investments in Digital Technologies: A Vision for Action in Digital Health.*

This Vision follows up from prior USAID policy, including the *Journey to Self-Reliance* and *Digital Strategy*, and interprets that guidance for the global health sector. It additionally maps out a path for the implementation of the *Principles of Donor Alignment for Digital Health*, which USAID co-authored and endorsed in 2018.

The *Vision* addresses the roadblocks of fragmentation, and lack of sustainability and interoperability, of many digital health technologies used in USAID's partner countries. To face these challenges the *Vision* highlights a systems-level approach to supporting partner countries' health sector digital transformation.

In support of this *Vision*, the policy document describes four priorities to guide related USAID planning, procurements, and programs. These are to assess and support:

- country digital health capacity,
- national digital health strategies,
- national digital health architecture, including where relevant through the use of global goods.

At its core, the Vision presents a roadmap for how USAID is able to strategically support its partner countries as they strengthen the digital transformation of their health sectors, especially by encouraging careful planning, interoperability, strong governance, and long-term sustainability.

Asia digital health information network

AeHIN was established following a conference in 2011 organized by WHO and USAID under the topics of health information systems interoperability. At the conclusion of the conference, participants were in agreement that health information system interoperability was lacking even within Ministries of Health. Three months later, the WHO hosted a second conference, with similar attendees reaching the same conclusions. The conferences delved in detail into the problems, but clear solutions did not arise. Frustrated with the stagnant state of affairs, a group of colleagues from Cambodia, Indonesia, Laos, Thailand, and Vietnam were gathered to work on common solutions to interoperability and to learn from each other's experiences.

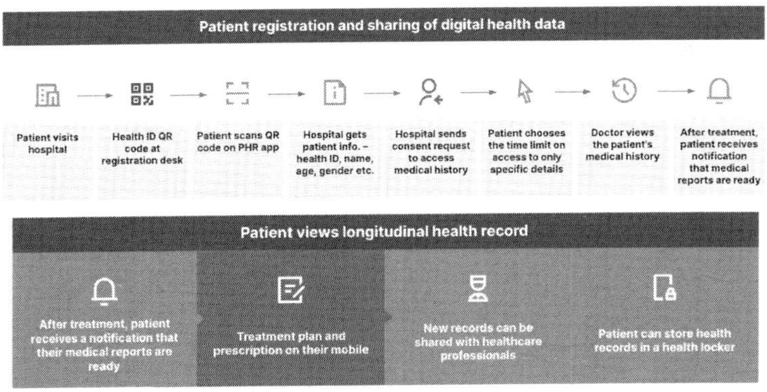

Figure 23. Patient-facing health records.

Source: Choudhury and Patil, 2021

With a small grant from WHO, seven colleagues from as many countries created AeHIN and developed a 5-year plan to develop the network. The network then received additional support from the Norwegian Agency for Development, USAID, and Canada's International Development Research Center to establish a platform for developing solutions. Following five annual meetings of the network, trusted relationships were developed that allowed members to assist each other in solving health information systems' interoperability issues. It is appreciated that the development partners, government representatives, and private-sector vendors who attend the annual meetings focus their discussions on how they can help countries in solving those problems.

The organization's main work has developed to connect with countries to address various gaps that are blocking interoperability. One common gap is not having a governance mechanism that can provide guidance for the activities of the many stakeholders and their competing agendas. As an example it is possible to get lost amidst the complexity of computerizing 1,600 hospitals in the Philippines, let alone one, without a framework and governance mechanism to guide them. Other important gaps are not having individuals with the right competencies and skills to build the architecture laid out in the framework and not having standards in place to create an interoperable architecture.

Assessment for Digital Health Competency Framework

The acquisition of competences must be ascertained as part of any training programme. Trainees from all the disparate specialities attending a digital health competency building program will have experience of both formative and summative processes that are created, and have been validated, to establish whether defined competences have been achieved. The most usual workplace based evaluations are developed for use within the clinical setting that the trainee is mostly working within and are unlikely hence to be immediately transferable for use with an eHealth framework. Similarly summative assessments including written standard examinations are designed to test the competences defined within the relevant specialty curricula.

The framework has defined the competences that ought to be acquired during an e-health training period but it is not within the remit of this framework to design new assessment tools. It is recommended, however, that a two-pronged process could be used to guarantee suitable assessment of trainees' competence acquisition. To begin with, as with the medical leadership framework, part of the existing workplace based assessments are able to be adapted to facilitate review of competence acquisition in eHealth. For example, the acute care assessment tool has features that make it suitable to use for assessing leadership competencies and assessments, including case based discussion. These could be similarly adjusted for use in e-health training.

Next, institutions making use of the framework, in collaboration with local educational centers could create a formal summative assessment based on the competences defined within this framework. For the latter evaluation this may be linked with the formal award of a diploma and thus may be the formal assessment of new knowledge, whereas the use of workplace based assessment would more suitably evaluate the application of skills and the relevant attitudes.

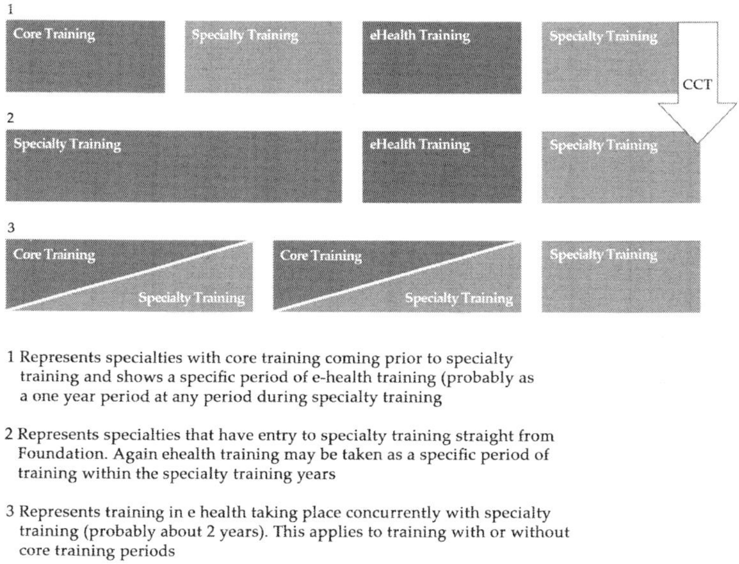

Figure 24. Representation of digital health training positioning.

Source: The Lancet Digital Health, 2022

Health Information Management

Exchanging health information in the context of a people-centric digital health ecosystem and with the intent of public interest should be championed with the user's consent, when pursued in a way that is built on trust, protects user privacy, secures digital systems, and guards against malign or inappropriate use. Such exchange is key as it may add to the enhancement of quality of processes, the results of health services and the ongoing care for patients (primary use of health data). It can additionally lead to the development of a knowledge base, which ought to be able to interact with other information systems including for example data on social determinants of health and registries.

The secondary application of health information is key to improve the quality of healthcare and research effectiveness. It could facilitate testing, validating and benchmarking artificial intelligence solutions and big data analyses across various parameters and settings, and the continuity of care of patients (primary use of health data). It also makes way for the construction of a knowledge base, which should be able to interact with other information systems, registries, etc. The secondary use of health information with appropriate de- anonymization of datasets would allow ethically managed testing, validating and benchmarking AI solutions and big data analyses across various parameters and settings.

Building Health Data Governance: Collecting, Protecting, and Sharing Data for Better Health Outcomes

Information lies at the core of digital health innovations. Nevertheless, health information is among the most strongly restricted forms of information (in regards to collection, use, sharing, and transferring). Health information does need specific attention as it covers sensitive personal information. Yet imposing overly harsh restrictions on its use does nothing to help optimize health outcomes. Policymakers in nations of all stages of development have not enforced or updated laws and regulations surrounding health data governance so that privacy and information protection challenges are addressed while guaranteeing there exists a clear framework for individuals, firms, and governments to exchange and utilize health data (in a protected and responsible way) to achieve its full potential. What this demonstrates is that there is a mismatch between policymakers (generally) seeing the potential of digital technologies—including for health—and how it needs changes to information governance frameworks. For example, WHO's 2015 *Atlas of eHealth Country Profiles* reports only 17 percent of respondents had a strategy to govern the use of information in the health sector.

The missing supportive health information governance frameworks surrounding the world comes at the center of an explosion in the range and volume of health information and services. The proliferation of wearables and other smart devices has significantly expanded the amount of user-generated health information (Shapiro et al., 2012). The ubiquity of mobile phones in LMICs has modified the situation for both health systems and individuals. Already, 1 in 10 mHealth applications have the ability to link to a sensor or device (Aitken and Lyle, 2015). These new technologies give opportunities to not only create, collect, and use large quantities of real-world data linked to health outcomes—defined as observational information obtained outside the context of randomized control trials and during clinical practice—but also make the delivery of new digital health services much cheaper and easier for a much broader range of users (FDA, 2020).

The following section looks at key challenges for health information governance: improving information collection, improving information protection, and facilitating access to health information.

Improving Health Data Collection

An information-driven approach to health governance is able to face one of a government's biggest hurdles: incomplete data. Digital health projects will be of minimal use if they lack the necessary information to start with, information coverage or information quality is limited, or they lack systems in place to maintain and improve on this information. It is thus paramount that nations, and their respective regulatory bodies and international workforces, include reasonable and responsible information collection efforts to ensure information is representative, complete, and applicable. The private sector has a role in assisting governments and their partners in comprehending the health of a community, including through public-private information exchange initiatives.

Country-wide governments, as well as their partners, must integrate health information collection into greater initiatives so as to better the institutional capacity of local agencies to gather information—in addition to undertaking health-specific steps to improve information gathering. The obstacle facing LMIC governments' traditional information gathering, such as national statistical offices and health agencies, is significant, as many of these agencies do not have resources and independence. Misaligned program incentives may additionally contribute to inaccurate information collection, among other factors (Jerving, 2019). Nevertheless, global agencies are teaming up to address this, including at the Partnership in Statistics for Development in the 21st Century and the Praia Group on Governance Statistics, in addition to the United Nations, the African Development Bank, and other multilateral agencies (Praia Group, 2020).

A suitable example is the Health Data Collaborative (HDC), a collective effort by global agencies, governments, donors, and academics to improve health information (HDC, 2018). HDC partners work with countries (such as Cameroon, Kenya, Malawi, and Tanzania) both to improve the availability, quality, and use of information for local decision-making and in recording progress toward the health-related Sustainable Development Goals (HDC, 2020). HDC shares a broad array of datasets, including data on routine health information systems, community data, facility surveys, measurement of quality of care, logistics management and information systems, disease surveillance, population data sources, household surveys, civil registrations, and other vital demographic statistics. HDC is creating a one-stop shop for health data system standards that will cover regulations for information collection, a standardized package of recommended indicators, data quality metrics, and other harmonized standards and survey tools (HDC, 2020).

Within information collection steps, it is also key to guarantee information collected is representative of the demographics. Doing so aids in facing the emerging "information divide"—the social and economic disparities that may be the outcome of a lack of collection or utilization of information regarding an individual or community. For digital health innovations to be of use, people, firms, academics, and governments must have access (within respective information privacy and protection regimes) to high-quality information about themselves and their communities. If some groups have no information collected about them, new discrepancies may come up as people in these populations are left outside digital health programs and interventions. In particular, policymakers may enact information gathering initiatives that target hard to-reach populations, ensure that funding programs targeted at closing the digital divide take into consideration the impact on information poverty, and help civic leaders in low-income regions understand the benefits of information and information gathering efforts.

Global information governance that permits the movement of health information and services across borders will be key to building an integrated and effective global digital health framework. Just as health conditions such as Ebola, malaria, and COVID-19 do not stop at national borders, health-care academics and providers must be able to effectively move information regarding these and other health obstacles across borders so as to prevent and manage them (Cory, 2020). The benefit of health information flows returns to the host nation in the form of better, faster, and more cost effective health services and results. Some examples of digital health campaigns that take advantage of the global flow of information include those such as Portal Telemedicina in Brazil, which utilizes cloud computing and AI to quicken diagnoses for users living in remote locations; and U.S.-Chinese partnerships in using AI and machine learning to accelerate the process of medicinal discovery.

Regardless of the significant advantages for companies, users, and national economies that come up from the capability of agencies to simply share information across borders, dozens of countries—across every stage of development—have risen barriers to cross-border information flows, including information-residency needs that strictly confine information within a country's borders (a concept known as "data localization") (Cory, 2017). Unfortunately, various countries have set up barriers to the exchange of health information. This stops companies from exchanging information overseas for analysis or service delivery—as companies usually depend on cloud-based IT systems to offer services for operations globally. Aside from explicit regulations for local information needs by mandating personal consent for cross-border transfers of information, thus making them harder and more expensive, if not impractical and impossible.

Some examples of set up and proposed information localization needs that affect health information and connected services are:

- In 2012, Australia set up the Personally Controlled Electronic Health Records Act, which requires individual health records be kept only in Australia (Personally Controlled Electronic Health Records 2012)
- Two Canadian provinces, British Columbia and Nova Scotia, have established regulations mandating individual information held by public bodies including schools, hospitals, and public agencies must be kept and accessed only in Canada, unless certain conditions are fulfilled (Chandler and Le, 2015).
- China has one of the widest collections of information localization policies globally, including for personal, financial, mapping, and health information. As of May 2019, China set up rules that not only force companies to keep genomic information locally, but also require all processing to take place locally and by local companies—as foreign organizations are explicitly banned from handling Chinese genomic data (National House Ordinance of the People's Republic of China, 2019).
- India's draft information protection bill allows the government to categorize any sensitive individual information as critical individual information and mandate its keeping and processing solely within India.This identifies the potential for localization, which would be matching with both India's recent decision to mandate localization for payments information and its

potential application for other types of information (Reserve Bank of India, 2018). Additionally, for other types of personal information, companies must keep a copy in India (known as data mirroring) prior to transferring data abroad (but only under certain conditions).

- In 2015, Russia passed a Personal Data Law that requires information operators that collect personal information about Russian residents must "record, systematize, accumulate, store, amend, update and retrieve" information using databases physically found in Russia (Morris, 2015).
- Nations also passed de facto barriers to transfers of health and genomic information that make it more difficult and more expensive, if not impractical, for firms to transfer it abroad. For example, South Korea and Turkey mandate that companies get explicit consent from residents in order to transfer sensitive information including genomic information abroad (Kim et al., 2018).

Certain policymakers utilize forced information localization policies in an erroneous attempt to achieve enhanced privacy or security. The location of information may impact how organizations answer lawful government requests for information. Yet controlling where agencies keep information does not affect how agencies gather and utilize information (privacy), or how they store and transmit the information (security). The notion that information must be kept domestically to guarantee it stays secure and private is mistaken. Regarding security, while some regulations may impose minimal security standards, the security of information does not depend on the nation in which data is kept, but rather only on the measures set up to keep it securely. In regards to privacy, information owners—whether they are individuals or businesses—depend on contracts and laws to limit voluntary information disclosures so information stored overseas receives the same level of protection as information stored domestically.

Communication

Healthcare is provided across several organizational set ups. Effective working in this interconnected healthcare environment needs clinical systems to communicate with each other reliably and safely.

Health care professionals must have a good grasp of the clinical systems and applications available to support user care and how to apply those applicable to their own practice. They should familiarize themselves with the role, functions and benefits of local systems and applications and must also understand the purpose and function of systems implemented at a country-wide level within their own nations.

Information technology is able to enhance clinical practice and new modes of working, including electronic order entry systems, Picture Archiving and Communication Systems (PACS) and electronic systems to enhance the management of medicines.

Clinicians must be aware of current and new technologies and how they can be applied in healthcare to enhance communication between healthcare professionals, users and carers, or to support more efficient and safe delivery of clinical practice. Technology may also be used for the identification of users, medicinal and blood products, lowering the risk of harm from administration to the incorrect recipient. Use of radiofrequency identification also allows agencies to manage their assets more efficiently.

Digital healthcare covers both digital health and telecare. Digital health refers to a range of initiatives targeted at providing improved, local and faster access to clinical services. Telecare supports beneficiary monitoring and management at home to lower admission rates to healthcare organizations and to allow self care and independence.

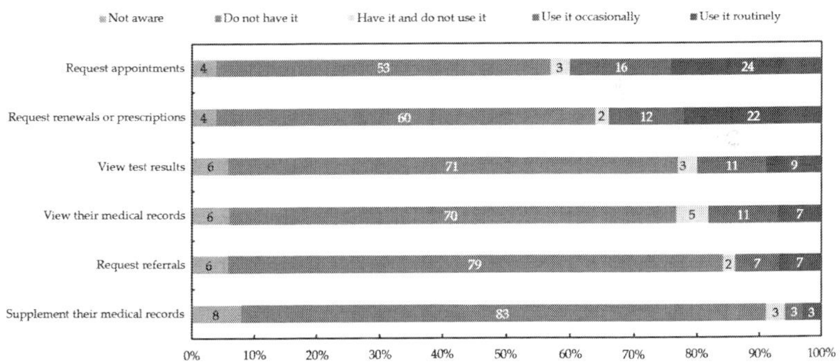

Figure 25. Functionalities available to patients in primary care medical records, as reported by the GPs.

Source: European Commission 2018

Professionalism

Professionalism represents the turning point for safe, effective and ethical health care activities. It gives priority to the welfare and well being of the user/client at its core, aligning with public expectations, guaranteeing it remains central in all clinical decisions and actions.

The information revolution of the last few years has modified several aspects of daily life. The Internet, e-mail, and numerous other technologies spew vast quantities of data with just a click of the mouse or a look at a personal organizer. Buried in the millions upon millions of Web sites are about 19,000 sites dedicated to the communication of health information. With so much health data so easily available, the following points must be considered:

How reliable is the information?

Will the data swap by e-mail remain confidential?

What policies are required to guarantee user safety?

The information revolution has not only provided a wealth of health information, but it has also set off changes in the patient-physician connection and in the notion of what it perceived as being a medical profession. Today, many physicians are against introducing new forms of connection into their practice. Of particular concern is many users'' desires to contact their health care providers via e-mail. While this would be a great convenience to users seeking routine answers such as appointments or test results, several doctors worry that they will be stormed by patients non-stop with incessant and often unreasonable petitions. Other doctors worry that patients may depend on email in situations that warrant an immediate response or even a visit to the emergency room or doctor's practice. In some cases, medical professionals have begun to add disclaimers to their own emails, informing recipients not to rely on e-mail communications if their message is urgent or sensitive.

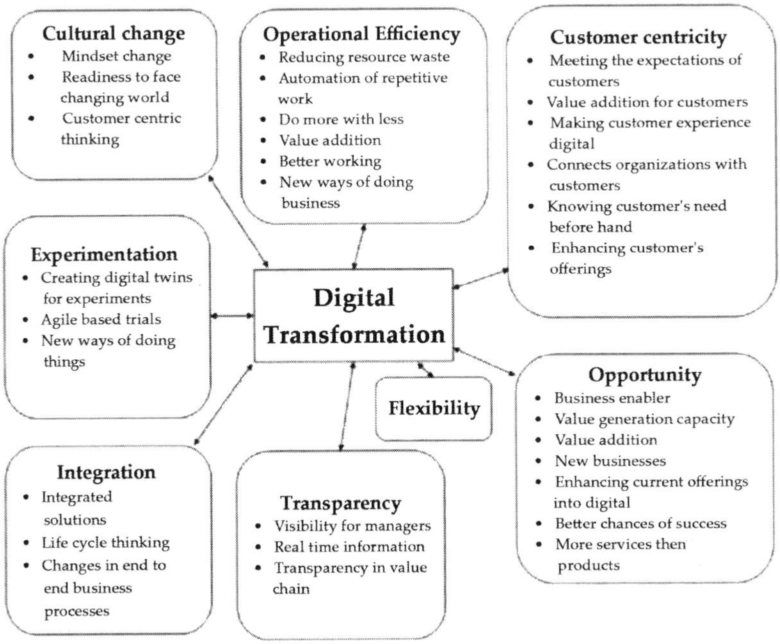

Figure 26. Conceptualization of digital transformation.

Source: Imran et al., 2021

Ironically, similar concerns were expressed upon the introduction of the telephone in the late 19th century. Several doctors thought that practicing medicine over the telephone compromised the moral integrity of the practice. Medical care providers were able to adjust to the use of the telephone by setting up answering machines and hiring secretaries. In an issue of the *Milbank Quarterly,* physician David Blumenthal states that doctors will be able to make the necessary changes to adapt to email. He goes on to state that, "if physicians are willing to accept some basic changes in their training, attitudes, and practices," then the information revolution will develop opportunities to not only preserve professionalism, but "enhance it."

The idea of professionalism is something that most people are cognisant of, but it is difficult to define. Paul Starr identifies 3 pillars of professionalism in *The Social Transformation of American Medicine*:

- The first is cognitive knowledge, the scientific knowledge and technical dexterity health care professionals have that allows them to diagnose and treat patients.

- Secondly, there is a moral component of professionalism, which requires that the needs of users come before the needs of the doctor.
- Finally there is a collegial responsibility for doctors to track and assess one another and to ensure competence in the profession. Collegial monitoring is peer-review and is necessary because the public does not know enough to evaluate the medical profession accurately.

Traditionally, the relationship between the physician and the patient was one-sided; meaning, doctors had vastly more information regarding medical conditions than their patients. This unbalanced distribution of knowledge made trust an integral part of a successful patient-doctor relationship. The medical profession's claim has been to provide "something that society cannot find elsewhere." The availability of health data on the internet severely reduces this claim by providing patients alternative sources for health management options. The question now is whether the information revolution will provide the public with sufficient knowledge to make decisions that were previously exclusive to doctors.

The information revolution can be thought of as a series of possibilities for increased connectivity between members of the health care system. The numerous links could cover superior communication between individual users, between patients and their doctors, and among doctors, patients, and healthcare facilities. This increased connectivity in the health care system will affect each of the 3 attributes that define professionalism.

Patients with internet access are able to search the web for huge quantities of information on a specific condition, whether it be through websites, or forums with other patients. Prior to a doctor's visit, a patient may have investigated possible diagnoses for his or her symptoms and may be cognisant of different management options. By assuming part of the physician's role, the patient effectively lowers the knowledge asymmetry in the patient-doctor relationship.

The multi-way communications may empower patient appreciation for the physician's moral commitment to prioritizing patients. Among the welter of patient-to-patient communication and of advertising on the internet and elsewhere, patients will find that it is only in the personal relation with their own health care providers that the information becomes tailored to them and their needs. This can happen only within the patient-physician relationship.

With increased connectivity, patients will possibly enter into the current system of self-governance that guarantees competence in the medical profession. They will be able to contact one another with greater ease, to compare and evaluate their visits to a particular practitioner. Perhaps more importantly, digital information already exists which focuses on evaluating specific hospitals on specific procedures, such as coronary bypass surgery, or back and neck surgery.

Information Systems and Technologies

Health records are utilized to provide a backup in patient care by acting as the repository of evidence for single clinicians, supporting clinical decision making and providing an important form of communication with other health care professionals and patients. They detail results of encounters with healthcare professionals and healthcare institutions. Health files give a legal account of care given and can be a source of information to support clinical audit, research, disease monitoring, service planning, allocation of resources and performance management.

Historically, health record keeping has been a clinician view of the activities between patient and clinician. To come, the record will turn into a shared enterprise with users directly accessing their full or partial information, which may contain not only a broader range of personal health, social and demographic information but also data and knowledge resources.

Open information policies are still rather novel and underused in LMICs. As an example, the progress of countries in sub-Saharan Africa toward enacting broad, consistent, and reliable open-data frameworks is slow overall and varied in practice (with cases of progression, but also regression, across the region) (Van Belle, 2018). Many countries lack the capacity, finances, or agreements to allow access to public and privately held information (Data Driven Development, 2015). Open information in many LMICs is also blocked by state-centric cultures within which it is considered enough to have public institutions alone holding, controlling and monitoring data information (African Development Working Group, 2014). Fortunately, LMIC policymakers have access to an increasing range of supra-national institutions (such as United Nations agencies, the World Bank, and the African Development Bank) and NGOs that provide resources and advice specifically on open information and related issues.

Policymakers can also try out new institutional models, including public-private partnerships, to improve information gathering activities and access. Governments can work in cooperation with private-sector companies on facilitating access to their specific country's information so as to increase understanding of their nation's residents, economy, and society—and their capacity to address public policy issues, such as in health. Nevertheless, this needs to be carried out on a voluntary basis, given forced access to information would otherwise undermine the commercial incentive for companies to develop and use information to begin with. Policymakers need to team up with private-sector companies to guarantee their proprietary, legal, and competition concerns are answered. Thus far, the set ups for sharing such proprietary information are not standardized, so private information in most existing public-private partnerships is just made available on an ad hoc basis.

Governing bodies, specifically public research institutions, are also able to encourage voluntary and mutually beneficial information sharing among private companies, researchers, and medical institutions—which may involve developing the technical architecture. As an example, the U.S. Department of Health and Human Services (HHS) announced a proposition of new guidelines that would facilitate access to user information by both patients and the health-care industry, in part by requiring the utilization of open application programming interfaces (APIs), which permits multiple software and databases to exchange information.

Governments may need to step in to encourage firms in particular areas to voluntarily share data. Although there is a net benefit from data sharing to patients and researchers, there is not always a short-term benefit to companies for making their data available to their competitors. A model effort is the Accelerating Medicines Partnership, a U.S. National Institute of Health-led drug discovery collaboration among 10 drug makers, wherein participating companies have created a shared database that exceeds the capabilities of any individual company's data holdings (Garde, 2014). Similarly, some pharmaceutical firms have recognized that sharing is in their collective interest and have participated in data-sharing programs, including the Accelerating Medicines Partnership and a GlaxoSmithKline-led initiative to share patient-level clinical trial data with other participating pharmaceutical companies (Kromholz, 2014). In other areas, such as medical device manufacturing, wherein data sharing has been a more difficult prospect, policymakers should conduct a review to identify factors preventing companies from sharing data with one another (Causey, 2014). And HHS recently announced proposed new rules that would facilitate access to patient data by both patients and the health-care industry, by mandating the use of open APIs.

Unfortunately, private-sector engagement in developing and creating these types of data-sharing frameworks and partnerships is very low in many LMICs. There are examples wherein private-sector firms help provide data-driven insights that support health outcomes, such as MedAfrica using open data to improve access to health information. Similarly, the cell phone company Orange has an open-data challenge "Data for Development (Blondel, 2013). Similarly, GovLab (based at New York University) helps different stakeholders—firms, research organizations, governments, and others—increase the availability and use of data by facilitating the exchange of data between different stakeholders. It has facilitated dozens of projects that involve health-related data.

Finally, policymakers should ensure patients themselves have access to the data they generate, and allow them to share it. At present, in most countries, there is no simple way for patients to contribute their personal data for use in medical research. This type of policy tool, similar to the Blue Button initiative for general health data in the United States, would give individuals insights into their own health and allow them to authorize third parties to create applications using that data, which holds the promise of helping their health in the future through better treatments.

These data-sharing efforts will help advance patient care in LMICs. Policymakers need to include these types of public and private data-sharing initiatives in their digital health strategies, as they will be crucial to achieving the end goal whereby respective parties can reasonably and responsibility access, share, and coordinate the full range of medical information—including medical histories, genomic data, behavioral data, and other sources—in order to provide better care to individual patients.

Patient Focus

Traditionally, healthcare data has centered around clinicians and institutions who largely controlled patient interaction. Lately, however, there has been a shift to consumer-centered systems. This is enabling patients to interact with health professionals and get involved in their own care, leading to greater engagement, improved outcomes and increased satisfaction.

Data about a patient is for the patient. A clinician is a custodian of the data, not the owner of the data, and that the patient or their authorized representative has a right to apply to see or obtain a copy of certain personal data held about them, including health records.

Clinicians should be able to provide informed support to patients on the range of online sources patients use to obtain information about their health, medical conditions and availability of services, including search engines, websites, discussion groups and social networks. Additionally, on the interactive services available to patients to support their healthcare needs, including (where available) online clinic booking, repeat prescriptions, and digital healthcare.

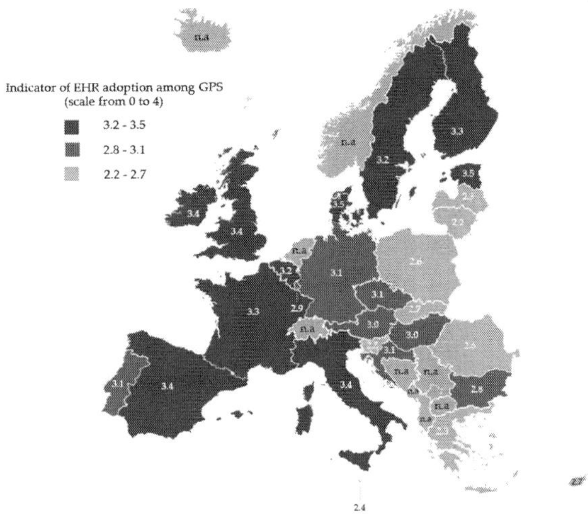

Figure 27. Electronic Health Record Adoption in the EU.

Source: European Commission 2018

A patient-focused approach to digital health competency building should allow for patient accessible electronic health records and patient held electronic personal health records of healthcare and empower them to become equal partners in the care process.

With instant access to a vast amount of healthcare information, tremendous opportunities exist to detect disease earlier, hasten the development of new treatments, and personalize them to individual patients. Connections between people, machines and data are set to further strengthen over the next decade thanks to advances in genetic engineering, next-generation semiconductors, machine learning and human-machine interfaces like biosensors and augmentation.

Emerging technologies in healthcare are changing the practice of medicine, and it can be difficult to stay current. As patients become more proficient in using digital devices, they have more opportunities to participate in their care. This means providers must consider the patient's experience at every stage in the continuum of care.

Patient-focused healthcare requires trusted partnerships between patients, providers, healthcare systems, and third-party payors.

In the early 2000s, person-centered care took the stage as providers and healthcare systems shifted away from the notion that a patient's role was simply to comply with physician orders. The person-centered approach has historically addressed chronic disease management in terms of episodic treatments, with a focus on the condition itself. In contrast, patient-focused care takes a more holistic view of how patients experience their medical conditions in the context of their daily lives. To achieve patient-focused care, patients and providers must build and maintain trusted, collaborative partnerships. This is what makes shared decision-making possible.

The foundation of patient-centered care is built on respect—respect for patient values, preferences, and choices about their health. To fully embrace a patient-focused care model, every treatment decision inside this model must be determined while viewing the patient as a unique individual.

Emerging technologies in healthcare delivery encourage patients to take an active role in their care, positioning them as directors rather than participants in their treatment journey. This flattens the hierarchy among members of the care team and promotes a spirit of equality where all voices are important within the continuum of care.

Multi-specialist medicine has to some degree undermined patient-focused care, fragmenting the patient experience and limiting the ability of providers to build long-standing relationships with patients. In this new patient-focused paradigm, successful health outcomes must be measured against patient personal goals *and* evidence-based guidelines. Providers cannot achieve desired outcomes without the patient's commitment and action.

Patient-Focused Healthcare Technologies

With the rapidly changing perception and adoption of digital technologies, patient-focused technologies augment traditional healthcare by improving patient engagement, satisfaction, and outcomes.

1. Digital Therapeutics (DTx)

Digital therapeutics are clinically validated technologies that treat, prevent, or manage medical conditions. Examples of digital therapeutics include wearables, such as heart rate monitors, activity trackers, blood glucose monitors, and pulse oximeters. The pharmaceutical industry is also exploring the use of software-based drugs.

DTx technology enables personalized medicine. For example, artificial pancreas systems integrate machine learning and artificial intelligence technologies to provide precise insulin dosages similar to that of the human pancreas. With digital health innovation, treatments are consistent, reducing the risk of human error and negative outcomes.

2. Telemedicine

Digital health grew deeper roots during the height of the COVID-19 pandemic, and experts expect the trend to continue as patients have come to value the convenience of telemedicine. One study found that 97.1% of patients and 100% of caregivers felt comfortable having sensitive and emotional conversations by video.

Telemedicine appears to have further growth potential, with some industry leaders considering it to be a digital form of personal protective equipment (PPE). Surgeons can also use telemedicine to extend their geographical reach since patients no longer need to travel long distances to complete follow-up visits after surgery.

Virtual care is a patient-focused approach that may also allow clinicians deeper insights into their patients' everyday lives.

3. Artificial Intelligence (AI)

AI is defined as "computer systems able to perform tasks normally requiring human intelligence." These innovative digital solutions include chatbots, robotics, virtual assistants, and other tools to identify and treat patients based on evidence-based algorithms. Using predictive analysis and pattern recognition technologies, patients receive timely, appropriate, and consistent treatment.

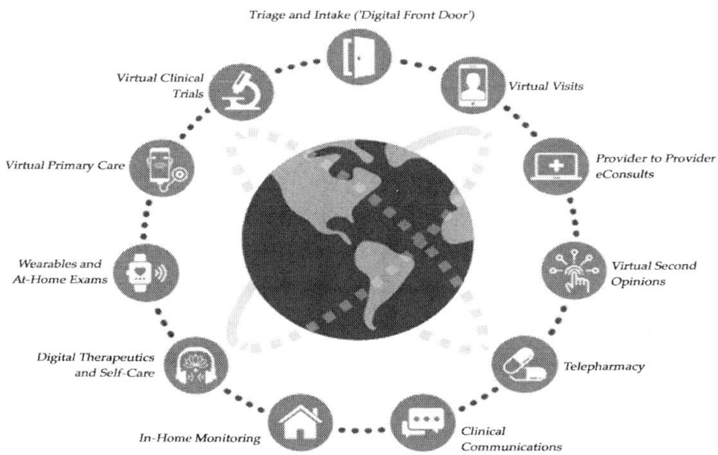

Figure 28. Digital Health Ecosystem.

Source: TripleTree, 2021

Health Analytics

The digital health framework, as identified above, is not intended to set a rigid pathway for digital health competency development, but rather to provide a key resource and common standards for the review, development, and alignment of profession-specific empowerment to ensure high-quality and consistent experiences. Attaining digital health competency will ideally involve embedding digital health within problem-based, case-based, and practice-based learning experiences and incorporate digital simulations and codesign projects. This work emphasizes core professional practice principles that underpin all activities involving digital health, including quality and safety, consumer-centeredness, critical thinking, and evidence-based practice.

As technologies evolve and practices involving digital health grow, it is critical to maintain attention to these core principles. The inclusion of performance cues within the framework provides a starting point to describe how successful competency might be demonstrated.

Although current health care professionals may now use digital technologies in their everyday work lives, they might have limited knowledge of the opportunities and issues that technology can bring to the health care landscape (Biggins et al., 2017). As a result, health care professionals require tailored opportunities to ensure that they develop or translate skills and knowledge to effectively practice in evolving digital workplaces.

Regular deployment and linking of health data for secondary purposes, such as to report on health systems performance, is increasingly adopted but relatively less common than the primary use of the data in the day-today provision of health services. Around a third of the countries report, for example, publishing of indicators on unplanned hospital readmissions, mortality at intervals after a given procedure, survival after diagnosis/ treatment, or appropriate prescribing of drugs (OECD, Forthcoming[5]).

The use of existing data to inform improvements in service delivery – through, for example, designing more tailored or better coordinated services – remains rare. While many countries pilot small projects aimed at an evidence-based redesign of health services, few implement new care models on a larger scale (OECD, 2019[8]). In Spain, for example, a locally developed risk stratification tool, exploring medical records data of primary care providers and hospitals, is used in 14 of the country's 17 autonomous regions. The tool is used to identify and group patients with complex care needs to improve targeting of care and allocation of healthsystem resources. The regions have built on this tool to tailor design integrated care models for each group of patients with complex care needs. Such models disencumber overburdened providers, for instance, by reducing unnecessary hospitalisations and the administrative workload of primary care physicians (OECD, 2019).

Moreover, there are also missed opportunities with regard to collecting data on patient reported outcomes (PROs) of care. As discussed above, digital technologies can help move away from reactive towards proactive approaches to preserving health by enabling greater participation of patients in the care process.

Digital Therapeutics

Digital Therapeutics covers a broad spectrum of digital tools integrated into clinical practice in support of normal therapy and care. It includes tools and systems used by clinicians within the provision of their interventions with patients, and varies from the use of online booking systems for scheduling, the identification and sharing of clinically-assured online health and care information, and specific tools relevant to the care provided.

This domain also covers the provision of remote care pathways (i.e. digital health, telemedicine, virtual care). Tools such as digital methods of data collection via mHealth apps or wearable technologies fall into this domain, as does the development, implementation and evaluation of remote care appointments via telephone or video.

Competencies include the user-led development and suitability of such services, as well as the evaluation of digital tools through the NICE Evidence standards framework for digital health technologies. Despite the wide spectrum of this domain, there is consensus across professions that this domain holds relevance across professions, irrespective of band.

Evolution of Frameworks

The digital health competency frameworks have drawn upon each other and have incrementally advanced the recommendations made in this area. The initial work of Staggers et al. (Staggers et al., 2001 and 2002), which targeted nurses at 4 levels of practice, has been reproduced and adapted to suit different nursing roles (eg, nurse leaders, nurse practitioners) (Curran, 2003; Westra et al., 2008), health professions (eg, dietitians) (Ayres et al., 2012), and even geographical settings (eg, Taiwan, Canada); (Nagle et al., 2014; Hwang et al., 2008). In another instance, to propose competencies for nurse leaders, Collins et al. (2017) expanded and reorganized competency categories from Westra and Delaney (Westra et al., 2008), which initially drew inspiration from the framework by Staggers et al. (Staggers et al., 2001 and 2002). The framework by Staggers et al. (2001 and 2002) was updated 10 years later by Chang et al. (Chang et al., 2011) with 42 new competencies.

Another commonly referenced framework is that by Egbert et al. (2016 and 2019). This framework identified 24 core competency areas and conducted a survey with experts to rank the most relevant competency areas for nurses in Austria, Switzerland, and Germany. The same survey with 24 core competency areas was then sent to multiple countries to put forth international recommendations for nursing informatics, widely known as the TIGER framework (Hübner et al., 2016 and 2018). The TIGER framework grouped the core competency areas into 6 overarching domains (ie, data, information and knowledge, information exchange and information sharing, ethics and legal issues, systems life cycle management, management in informatics, biostatistics, and medical technology) and ranked the most relevant competencies for nursing internationally. Subsequently, the TIGER framework prompted its 2.0 version to include a wider spectrum of healthcare workers (Hübner et al., 2019) and inspired the work by Thye et al. (2018) where interprofessional competencies were identified.

One framework that was accessible through an open-source internet-based database is the HITCOMP Tool and Repository (2002). HITCOMP was produced by the eHealth Workforce Development Workgroup as part of the EU*US eHealth Work Project. Its overall goal was to map, quantify, and project the needs of a digitally competent workforce (Technology Informatics Guiding Education Reform, 2017). This tool covers the digital competencies required in acute care settings for 5 broad roles of health care workers, similar to the TIGER framework version 2.0 (ie, direct patient care; administration; engineering or information, communication, and technology; informatics; and research or biomedicine) (Hübner, 2019). In comparison with the other included frameworks, the HITCOMP framework has the highest number of competencies at 1025. Other frameworks that inspired the development of subsequent frameworks include the IMIA (Mantas et al., 2010), which was adapted by the AHIEC (Australian Health Informatics Education Council, 2011) to create national informatics standards for Australian health professionals, health informaticians, and specialists; the frameworks by Barakat et al (2013) and the Academy of Medical Royal Colleges (Academy of Medical Royal Colleges, 2011), which were adapted by Van Houwelingen et al. (2016) to develop a digital health framework aimed at nurses; and the telepsychiatry framework by Hilty et al. (2015), which laid the foundation for telebehavioral health competencies by Maheu et al. (Maheu et al., 2018).

THE IMPACT OF GOVERNMENTAL AND HEALTH CARE PROFESSIONALS' INVOLVEMENT FOR DIGITAL HEALTH COMPETENCY DEVELOPMENT

Given the inherent nature of digital health as being innovative and transformative, it is critical that the health care workforce becomes suitably prepared and adaptable to these available and wide ranging tools. Tertiary education of future health care graduates needs to move from a focus on technical skills to encompass broader digital health competencies.

Developing digital health competencies extends beyond technical proficiency to include the integration of technology into current practice and demonstrating a strong ethos around lifelong learning and transforming care. By re-evaluating traditional resources used in education and incorporating knowledge around digital health competencies, educational curriculum will provide greater opportunities to build capability in working with systems undergoing digital transformation (Gray et al., 2016).

Consistent with previous research (Li et al, 2017; Gray et al., 2014) it has been possible to identify the need for educational development to reinforce existing digital health competencies, adapt existing capabilities to make them transferable to novel contexts, and introduce new learning opportunities for interactions with technologies within education and practice encounters. In essence, developing digital health competencies assists in bridging the gap between academia and the application of digital health by emerging and existing health care professionals.

Digital health technologies are changing the way health and care are delivered, reshaping medical practice and the patient-doctor relationship. Digital health literacy (DHL) of healthcare professionals is a crucial component of the efficient and effective transformation of healthcare. Doctors should possess strong digital skills framed and adapted to their medical specialty.

At present, neither the practicing health professionals nor the generation in training are adequately prepared. Doctors need to be involved in the early stages of the development of digital solutions and understand technologies' limitations to form realistic expectations and reduce misconceptions about their role and usefulness. They need to ensure appropriate professional oversight over clinical validation, while remaining conscious of the overreliance of technology.

Below are some examples of national digital health initiatives around the World.

Denmark

The third happiest country in the universe has one of the most advanced digital health systems alongside an elaborated and concise national digital health strategy for the next four years. The document emphasizes the importance of the cooperation of each and every healthcare actor through the easiest and fastest way, technology, with a clear purpose: to build an integrated network focusing on patients and looking at the person as a whole, not just at the individual diagnosis.

Pros. Denmark is building a robust digital system with enhanced safety for patient data as well as a framework for coordination among platforms and actors. Currently, a patient's medical records are viewable by clinicians across regions in the National Health Record (Sundhedsjournalen). In addition, the Shared Medication Record (Fælles Medicinkort) gives healthcare professionals access to a complete, up-to-date prescription-medicine overview for the patient across the entire health system. The massive digital system enables Danish GPs, health facilities, nursing homes and other facilities to cooperate better and decrease inequalities.

As another building block of digital health, the Danish government encourages the arrival of empowered patients on the scene alongside with more focus on prevention. With acknowledging the projections for growth in chronic illnesses while being aware of strained resources, the document outlines the importance of patients taking an active role in their care: to understand their data and their medical state better, and furthermore to proactively participate in their treatment. That also means a shift towards prevention.

Cons. The Medical Futurist has to say, we couldn't find a single flaw in the strategy! We are enthusiastic about the clear vision and well-thought-out steps of the Danish government, which hold up an excellent example of how policy-makers should approach digital health.

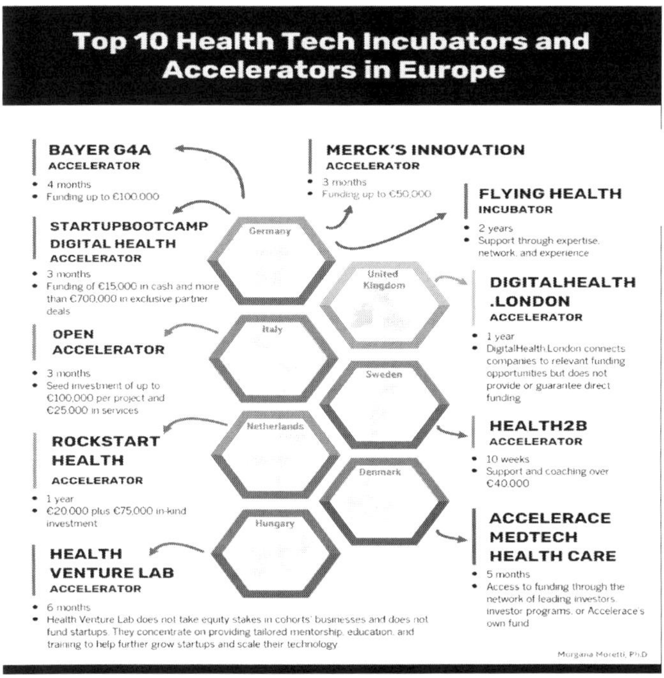

Figure 29. Top health tech incubators and accelerator in Europe.

Source: Moretti, 2021

Australia

The country recognized two years ago that it needs a digital health strategy, so Canberra established the Australian Digital Health Agency and consulted every stakeholder in the healthcare landscape. The forums, workshops, webcasts and town hall meetings were attended by more than 3,100 people, and over 1,000 submitted their recommendations. Thus, drawing up the Australian digital health strategy was an entirely inclusive process.

Pros. The result is a document focusing on leveraging on a digitally savvy society and directing it towards a crystal-clear digital health vision with patients put in the center of care. It says that by the end of 2018, every Australian will have a My Health Record unless they choose not to. By 2022, all healthcare providers will be able to contribute to and use health information in My Health Record on behalf of their patients, while they will be able to access their health information at any time online and through mobile apps. The strategy outlines the goals to improve patient pathways and the overall patient experience, sustain a more efficient health system, provide greater access to care and at the same time full data security.

Cons. The strategy places its focus too much on health IT challenges such as electronic medical records, personal health records or interoperability, while cultural transformation and its consequences such as patient engagement, dealing with patient data as well as the utilization of health sensors get a lower priority.

New Zealand

In 2016, the Health Ministry of New Zealand also realized that *the health sector will need to be adaptable in the coming years as developing technology changes how services can be delivered in ways not yet understood*. So, they started to think strategically about how they could ensure that all New Zealanders "live well, stay well and get well" in a patient-centered healthcare ecosystem. The government prepared the NZ Health Strategy with the aim to transform the existing processes and practices so that they align with 21st-century challenges, and launched a mechanism to build their digital health strategy embedded in the framework.

It means they want to have a greater focus on people and their needs while including everyone in shaping healthcare processes together. On the other side, they want to create an integrated healthcare system that provides comprehensive services. They worked out five central elements to define the

NZ system: people-powered, closer to home, value and high performance, one team, and a smart ecosystem.

Pros. The vision is entirely patient-centered, inclusive and forward-looking. Moreover, the Medical Futurist was honored that the New Zealand government reached out to our team for advice, and they included the definition of digital health worked out by The Medical Futurist Institute in their latest draft version of the digital health strategy.

Cons. The strategy in its current form is only a draft which still needs to be approved by the Director of General Health. Thus the country hasn't initiated any of the major changes that the strategy promises.

Israel

The small country is one of the biggest players in digital health in the Middle East. In March 2018, the Israeli government announced that it will invest $275mn in its digital health strategy. In July, Jerusalem announced a $33 million grant aimed at furthering the country's foothold in biotech and medicine. Thus, it is clear that the state is ready to invest in the digital health scene, which is a definite upside.

Pros. According to the document itself, the primary goal of the digital health strategy is to unify the existing database of the digital medical records Israel has collected throughout 20 years — which holds the medical files of more than 98 percent of the population. Furthermore, it aims to create a single database, in which one's participation is optional, which will help attract researchers and industry leaders from across the globe. Beyond that, the government aims to strengthen telemedicine, to facilitate collaboration between various institutions providing care and to improve emergency rooms.

Cons. Although the digital health strategy mentions the word proactivity, it is not used regarding urging patients to proactively take care of their own health. What's more problematic, though, that the holistic approach, as well as the central values of digital health such as the patient-doctor partnership and the democratization of care, are entirely missing.

Rwanda

In the last couple of years, massive health reforms were introduced in the African country. However, a digital health strategy has not taken shape yet.

Rwanda introduced electronic health records for HIV services in partnership with intergovernmental organizations, WHO, Global Fund, OCDC or the US Government. Then they expanded the EHR system to manage financial aspects, registration, consultation, clinical records, etc. Currently, they are using an e-LMIS for the management of medical supplies, lab management systems for logistics in laboratories and a rapid SMS system. Using the latter, the approximately 60,000 community health workers in the country can report about any emergency to the Health Ministry in a short time.

Pros. The government is saying that at the moment, they are integrating all the various systems together, and approximately within the next ten years, the Rwandan medical landscape will be completely transformed with a strong focus on digital health. These are not empty phrases, health start-ups are flocking to the country after positive experiences of companies such as Babylon Health or Zipline.

Cons. No unified document outlines the digital health strategy of Rwanda for the next couple of years.

Nigeria

In 2013, the Nigerian Minister of State for Health looked at the national health landscape, and he was convinced that technology could be leveraged to impact health outcomes but was concerned by the abysmally low return on investment given the huge amounts of money being put into technology in the health sector, said Olasupo Oyedepo. Working with the communication technology minister, the Minister of State for Health secured support from the Norwegian Aid Agency through the United Nations Foundation and created a process and project—tagged ICT4Saving One Million Lives—to, among other things, drive the development of a national eHealth strategy. Oyedepo recounted that the strategy development team ran into a number of problems. The first problem, which many low- and middle-income countries (LMICs) experience, is that any digital health strategy needs to be designed with the end users in mind, but the intended end users were not appropriately informed about digital health to provide useful input. Thanks to the flexibility of their donor, Oyedepo and his colleagues were able to take 3 months to focus on educating stakeholders about the digital health ecosystem. They also used the World Health Organization (WHO) and International Telecommunication Union national strategy document as a guide and invested time strengthening and building the capacity of the digital health ecosystem.

These efforts paid off, said Oyedepo, because the resulting conversations with potential partners in government, the private sector, international development organizations, and the health sector became more than just listening to presentations and taking notes. "We had individuals in the room who could drive a discussion about how digital [strategies] will really help optimize health," said Oyedepo. The lesson here, he said, was "strengthen the capacity of the group you are working with and life becomes easier." Instead of driving the conversation, his team's major job was to keep people on track, document ideas, and help tease out the substance of those ideas.

The vision of the resulting national health strategy is that by 2020, eHealth will help enable and deliver universal health coverage in Nigeria. Arriving at that vision, he recalled, involved many heated discussions. Some of the stakeholders wanted the focus to be on affordability, others on improving access to care and the quality of care, but in the end, everyone realized that all of these are attributes of universal health coverage.

The purpose of Nigeria's national digital health strategy was to put in place overarching guidance for the use of technology in health and to then strengthen the capacity of the necessary and appropriate government structures to govern the implementation of proven technologies throughout the nation. Today, Oyedepo and his colleagues are working to support the government's efforts to create and strengthen those governance structures, build capacity, strengthen collaborations, and empower the government to be able to ask some fundamental questions before it makes digital health investments that best serve Nigeria's needs and that can be sustainable when outside funding ends.

One lesson he has learned over the course of these activities has been that when putting together partnerships, whether with donor organizations, governments, or the private sector, it is essential to acknowledge the role, value, and relevance of every partner. For example, there is nothing wrong with a private company wanting to make a profit or with government wanting to improve the lifestyle of its citizens. The key is to find the middle ground that reflects the values important to each partner. Finding that middle ground depends more on the people and organizations involved than the technology, and it requires building trust and a strong sense of collective ownership among the partners.

For a governance structure, the network has adopted the COBIT 5 framework developed by the Information Systems Audit and Control Association, and 22 people from network countries have become framework certified. Marcelo said that these individuals now have the confidence that they can manage the complexity involved in creating and managing an interoperable, nationwide eHealth information system. Regarding system architecture training, the network has adopted The Open Group Architecture Forum (TOGAF) certification framework, and there are now 12 certified enterprise architects in Asian ministries of health. He explained that those who passed were health professionals, not technical staff. Later, this group of architects reviewed and adopted the Open Health Information Exchange (OpenHIE) interoperability framework as one with just enough sophistication and complexity for LMICs to understand and implement, said Marcelo.

Currently, the network is working on developing program management skills among network members, and the Malaysian Ministry of Health is offering a training program that includes planning, procurement, program evaluation, and monitoring. The network is also looking at the PRINCE2 (Projects In Controlled Environments) and PMP (Project Management Professional) frameworks for program management. Marcelo noted that once network countries have developed capabilities in governance, architecture, and program management, they will be able to select among the many standards that exist for interoperability.

PPPs can only develop and be successful when the government realizes that it has to do its part, which is developing those capabilities. With a governance structure, architecture, and program management capabilities in place, private-sector companies can then come in with their technologies and data and create national health information systems that are interoperable. He noted, though, that governments already have relationships with companies in the private sector that have developed from technology acquisition programs outside of the health sector, and that these relationships can be important when the health ministry starts talking to vendors about purchasing technologies. In fact, the network holds a biweekly webinar during which ministries of health and national insurance agencies talk about how they were able to solve specific problems working with specific vendors, who when asked, are allowed to discuss the features that enabled a particular solution. “We decided it will be the ministry making the presentation and the private-sector vendor providing support to the ministry,” said Marcelo. “I think that is a good way to model public–private partnerships, where the government shows leadership and the private sector shows support.” As a final comment, he said AeHIN is starting to work with countries in Africa and hopes to start a collaboration soon with Oyedepo's group in Nigeria, which is also certifying people in COBIT 5.

Why do countries need a digital health strategy at the national level?

Building up a digital health strategy would mean the reasonable regulation of options for patients opened up by technological solutions. The digitization of healthcare as well as other parts of society entails transnationalization and the disappearance of boundaries. Cross-border cooperation in healthcare through technologies could enable treatments outside the scope of the national healthcare systems – which was unimaginable before. It might happen already today that someone receives state-of-the-art care without crossing the threshold of any hospital in his own country.

Imagine that a patient living in France asks a Belgian company to sequence the tissue of his tumor. Afterward, another enterprise in precision diagnostics establishes that a Swiss pharma company has precisely that type of clinical trial on a Spanish island, which the patient could use – for free. In case, the treatment proves to be effective, the person will be healed without the expertise of French doctors. Thus, why exactly would he contribute to the healthcare system through his taxes in France? Governments could avoid the appearance of such future scenarios with the careful crafting of national digital health strategies.

CHAPTER 2

GOVERNMENTAL ROLE IN THE DEVELOPMENT OF DIGITAL HEALTH COMPETENCIES

CONTENTS

While digital technology can improve health outcomes, particularly in low-resource settings, a fragmented landscape of actors and interests working to implement digital health solutions can lead to a lack of coordination, waste, and unrealized benefits. There can be an opportunity to build health solutions around market needs in a coordinated and integrated way if digital health strategies are aligned with the health priorities established by countries and communities. Starting with country- and community-led priorities can aid the private sector in developing digital health strategies that are responsive to the needs of patients and communities. Collaboration among the actors of the ecosystems for health and technology advances the opportunities for business and therefore impact.

Clinicians contributing to eHealth at a local or national level need to be aware of the organizational, economic and political context. This requires an understanding of health service delivery, both local and national, and how eHealth initiatives support the strategic direction of travel and contribute towards improving business processes.

The approval of regulatory paths for digital health, which have spread from the US to Europe in France, UK and Germany, are expected to increase the number of patients and physicians experiencing the availability of new approaches and options in their care pathways. One of the major challenges of the upcoming years will therefore be to enhance the awareness and understanding of digital health (that is, boost digital health literacy) among the various stakeholders, thus creating the conditions for proper adoption.

As in other fields of innovation, the adoption process in the digital healthcare space appears to follow a 'pulled' rather than a 'pushed' route, driven by technology that rapidly generates applications and need-driven interactions.

Digital-solution providers and governments often have interlocking relationships when deploying large-scale solutions. In settings in which governments and nongovernmental organizations are ill equipped to build and deploy solutions on their own, technology innovators have a critical role to play. Solution providers can evaluate how to integrate with government systems and may depend on strong, top-level government leaders to champion system change and drive user adoption.

It is important to establish relationships and credibility with other trusted and already-established stakeholders at an early stage. Partnering with established organizations, service providers, or government agencies is often vital to reaching scale. In Kenya, for example, foundational in-country partnerships established prior to the COVID-19 pandemic leveraged the partners' deep market understanding and consumer experience. To date, M-TIBA, a financial-technology platform, has connected more than four million users and 1,200 healthcare providers in Kenya.

Other examples of partnerships among governments and digital-solution providers include Turn.io's chatbot app, which allowed more than 11 million symptom checks in South Africa, and the Vietnam Ministry of Health's launch of a suite of digital tools, including NCOVI and Bluezone, to respond to the pandemic. As of March 2021, Bluezone had been downloaded by 24.2 percent of the population, and NCOVI had been downloaded by 19.8 percent of the population, allowing users to receive critical health information during infection spikes.

The current digital-primary-healthcare landscapes of most LMICs are characterized by fragmented solutions, with some examples of national-level excellence along a single healthcare journey. Depending on their current state, LMICs could aspire toward one of three end states in digital primary healthcare :

- interoperability among multiple healthcare journeys at national level
- a national healthcare ecosystem that connects all healthcare journeys and patient data
- regional interoperability and integration on key use cases, such as cross-border public-health surveillance

Prioritizing a national healthcare ecosystem can enable data flow and foster collaboration among key stakeholders to achieve the following improvements:

- Expansion of healthcare coverage. Expansion could allow broader reach of healthcare delivery through technological solutions.
- Enhanced quality of services. Better-quality services could support improved coordination of care through data sharing and provide a convenient and seamless user experience. They could also enhance the quality of professionals, providing data and analytics for evidence-based guidelines.
- Resource optimization. Optimization could enable earlier detection of risks through predictive analytics and enable long-term cost management. In the near term, it could also have a significant impact on management efficiency by allowing increased division

of labor and overall utilization through centralized, coordinated, real-time management.

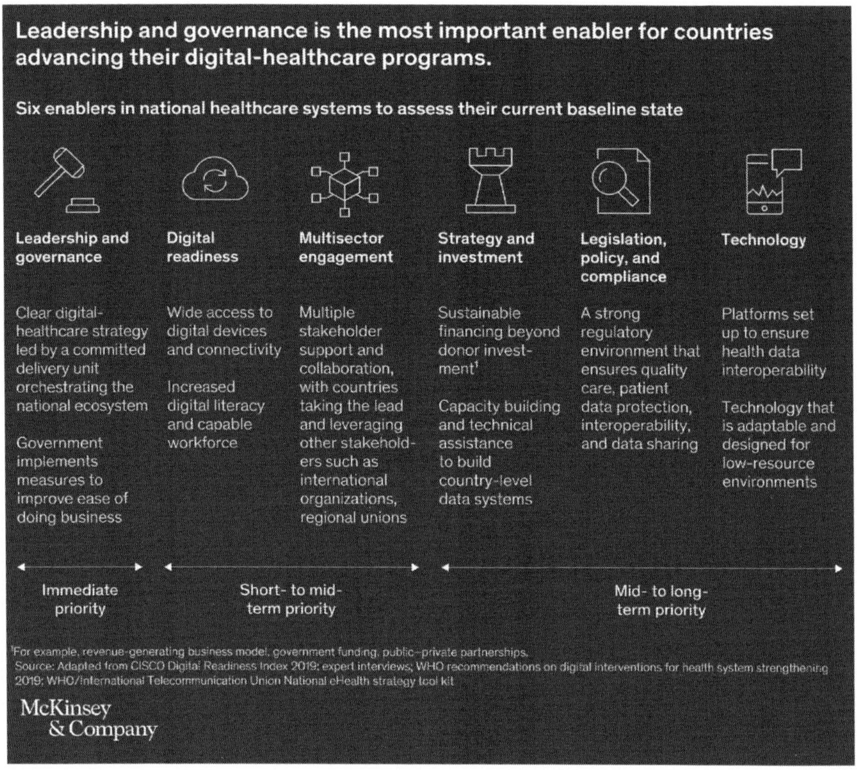

Figure 30. Enablers in national healthcare systems.

Source: McKinsey & Company, 2021

WHY DOES EVERY COUNTRY NEED A DIGITAL HEALTH STRATEGY?

Three reasons necessitate the urgent introduction of a digital health strategy in every country.

(1) First and foremost, healthcare systems are unsustainable. According to OECD projections, in Europe, public expenditure on health and long-term care in OECD countries is set to increase from around 6% of GDP today to almost 9% of GDP in 2030 and as much as 14% by 2060. The international organization

also found that the causes for the rising public costs stem from the growing needs of aging populations, the increasing share of chronic illnesses in societies, the rising incomes driving higher expectations – and the introduction of new technologies.

(2) Secondly, the needs-based shortage of healthcare workers globally is about 17.4 million, says The Medical Futurist Institute in its latest paper. That's almost the entire population of Chile and twice as many as living in Austria or Israel. Moreover, the WHO's *Global Strategy on Human Resources for Health: Workforce 2030* reports that shortages can mount up to 9.9 million physicians, nurses and midwives globally by 2030.

(3) Thirdly, technology is outpacing healthcare systems as well as bureaucratic authorization systems at lightning speed. The market of digital health technologies, including health IT, wearables, health sensors and any solutions aiming to digitize healthcare, is projected to surpass USD 379 billion by 2024; according to a research report by Global Market Insights published in April 2018. Investment is pouring into the sector as never seen before: Rock Health reported that at the close of its third quarter, 2018 is already the most-funded year ever for digital health startups.

Thus, every national government needs a digital health strategy to be able to channel the power of health technologies to tackle the human resources crisis as well as to make healthcare systems sustainable. We need digital health for both.

NATIONAL DIGITAL HEALTH STRATEGIES

Developing a national digital health strategy is a critical first step for identifying, prioritizing, and addressing barriers and shortfalls in key enablers for digital health. A comprehensive local assessment is crucial to developing a long-term plan, coordinating with development and other partners, and mobilizing the political support necessary for resourcing and implementation.

An effective digital health strategy requires leadership and buy-in from federal (and regional) governments, supported by representatives from all relevant government agencies and non government stakeholders, including the private sector, nonprofit organizations, and overseas development agencies. A whole-of-government approach is needed as health agencies cannot operate in a silo disconnected from ICT, economic, science, health, and innovation agencies, as well as data privacy and protection agencies.

Proper financial support is essential, especially given new programs and technologies will be layered on top of existing IT systems and organizational structures, which often means significant up-front costs. This also highlights the need for governments, development partners, and other stakeholders to invest in coordinated plans rather than ad hoc projects and policies. Unfortunately, many LMICs have already succumbed to the latter approach and face a proliferation of uncoordinated digital health projects, which is more likely to lead to unsustainable and ineffective uses of digital health tools.

Box 15. Leveraging data to improve surveillance

Global health emergencies bring strongly to light the importance of comprehensive, comparable, and uptodate data within and between countries. If deployed well, digital technologies and interconnection provide access to such data and can help to better detect, monitor, comprehend, respond to, and recover from crises such as the COVID19 pandemics.

Countries with standardized national EHRs can, for example, follow up much more comprehensively on the full spectrum of health outcomes, in addition to the incidence and death rates. However, as discussed above, most countries do not have the technical and operational readiness to generate such information from EHRs (OECD, 2020).

Countries with low interconnection between data systems had to embark on ad hoc efforts to quickly gather data on, for example, treatments and outcomes of patients with COVID19 to help providers in learning about and adopting best practices. In Germany, for example, an initiative to create a unified record of all COVID19 patients treated across all German university hospitals has been launched within a matter of days, with quick deployment of funding for this project by the Ministry of Research (Federal Ministry of Education and Research, 2020).

Furthermore, realtime administrative data on, for example, hospital bed capacity at a regional or national level is of high value. Only a few countries, such as Denmark and Sweden, have systems allowing for monitoring hospital bed capacity, including in intensive care units (ICUs), with acceptable time lag. These systems allow for more precise responses to capacity constraints in situations such as a pandemia. In other countries, Germany, for example, in the face of COVID19 outbreak, the Robert Koch Institute (RKI), the German Hospital Association (DKG), and the German Association of Intensive and Emergency Care (DIVI) together have set up within days a new website where each hospital can update daily their available capacity for intensive care with respiratory support (DIVI, 2020). Similarly, a centralized system to which hospitals provide daily data on bed occupancy, both in critical and conventional care, has been established rapidly in Spain.

While many countries have recognized the importance of national digital health strategies, there are significant gaps in many regions around the world. WHO's 2015 survey of eHealth policies revealed that 72 countries (58 percent) of the 125 member countries (that responded) have defined national digital health strategies and corresponding plans to implement them. Notable exceptions include Brazil, India, Indonesia, and Mexico. The Global Digital Health Index observes that Malaysia, the Philippines, and Jordan are well advanced in this area, with fully costed national plans currently being implemented. Malaysia in particular is lauded for its integrated digital health strategy, which has been ongoing for 15 years and is linked to the national 5-year rolling Malaysia Plans for social and economic transformation.

Thankfully, international agencies are working to help countries that have yet to develop a national strategy. For example, WHO's International Telecommunications Union (ITU) National E-Health Strategy Toolkit aims to assist member states in the development and implementation of digital health policies and strategies, and subsequent integration with their national health-care systems. The toolkit is an expert, practical guide that provides a solid foundation and method for developing and implementing a national digital health vision, action plan, and monitoring framework.

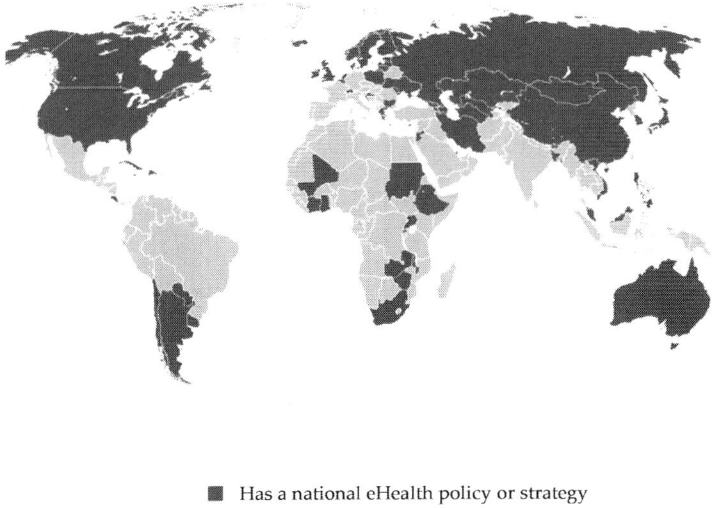

Figure 31. Countries with national eHealth policies or strategies.

Source: WHO, 2015

Governments Need to Provide Foundations for Trustworthy, Ethical, and Human Centered Digital Transformation

Providing leadership with an overarching and human centric digital health strategy

A successful digital transformation amounts to a health systemwide reorganization, and, as such, it requires leadership with an overarching strategy that articulates how technology driven innovation strengthens health systems and forms a framework for coordination among all the decision making actors, where the parties agree to continuously prioritize specific initiatives. A good digital strategy illustrates how digital technologies can provide solutions to problems that health workers encounter in their daily jobs; in particular, it defines focus areas for achieving the objectives of putting patient needs first and making daily workflows easier.

The strategy should also form a part of a broader cross-sectoral digital strategy in order to support joint initiatives in the areas where there are interdependencies across different sectors, such as health and education.

Advancing evaluation and regulatory safeguards to ensure positive impact of digital technologies

The transformative potential of digital technologies implies huge prospective benefits but also risks and the possible diversion of resources to ineffective digital tools. Hence, their implementation needs to be accompanied by robust evaluation and monitoring to assess their true impact on prevention and health care. This is particularly the case for more disruptive technologies, such as Artificial Intelligence, for which knowledge about the consequences is limited when first implemented and any undesired effects cannot be fully anticipated and averted. Once a technology is widely used, the consequences become known, but it might be difficult to adapt the technology or the legal and organizational environment to timely counteract any undesired effects.

Depending on the technology, there are two solutions to the above problems:

- to increase knowledge of benefits and risks at initial stages of the development and use of a new digital technology. This can be realized through advancing the methods for systematic evaluation of the impact of digital health technologies, which, at present, are largely based on methods primarily developed and used for pharmaceuticals

- to increase social control over technological trajectories through regulatory safeguards and monitoring for digital technologies, Artificial Intelligence in particular, during their lifetime.

Promoting user friendly design of digital technologies

The usability of digital technologies is one of the major drivers of the adoption. Yet, the experience to date shows numerous examples of technologies that instead of aiding the work of health professionals, get in its way. Most challenges result from a failure to adequately engage end users in the design process and understand the complexity of work in health care, despite the existence of well developed methods that can aid such engagement and understanding.

Hence, there is a need to further strengthen regulations regarding technology design, such that producers face incentives to meaningfully engage with the end users and the public procurement of digital tools and solutions includes user friendliness among the selection criteria. Countries can also consider issuing guidelines for the producers or collecting information on user experience with digital technologies to improve knowledge of problems and inform work on improvements.

Human expertise and skills need to be advanced to enable digital technologies to add value

Digital health is frequently only available as an elective course in education or professional training programmes and not taught at a high enough level. Moreover, it is presented as a standalone subject rather than being integrated across subjects, which is not conducive to building a digital culture or the perception of digital technologies as an integral component of health services.

This calls for ensuring the presence of digital health in the core content of education and professional training as well as investment in creating modern and comprehensive digital health curricula for future and current health workers. The curricula should not only focus on skills for merely operating digital tools, but also on skills such as critical appraisal of information and digital health ethics.

To meet the current demand for digital upskilling more systematic support should be created that ensures upskilling for all categories of health workers, in particular through more flexible (self) learning opportunities. The prevailing problems of Continuous Professional Development (CPD) and other professional training systems, such as a lack of dedicated time or means for upskilling on the part of health workers, need to be also addressed.

Merging of 'hightech' and 'hightouch' skills

While digital technologies have allowed for means of social connection that have not been possible before, they can also often cause a deterioration in the quality of social interaction. Therefore, the development of specific interpersonal skills, particularly in patient centered communication and shared patient provider decision making, needs to be further emphasized in health education and training.

Moreover, experience from other industries illustrates that the emerging digital tools based on developments in Artificial Intelligence will require skills in counteracting automation bias, i.e. the phenomenon of favoring suggestions made by automated systems, while ignoring other sources of information. The health education sector needs to acknowledge this problem and invest in work on training devised to tackle it.

Creating a larger cadre of individuals with hybrid skill mix to manage the transformation

Addressing the critical challenges of digital transformation requires policy makers and technologists as well as clinical leaders/managers and technologists to work together and understand more of each other's fields. However, health systems lack clinician leaders and managers with a combined understanding of clinical practice, technology, and change management. There is also evidence of a deficit of informaticians and system optimisers with strong insights into health care.

This requires more of the joint degree and hybrid educational programmes that combine the understanding of, for example, clinical practice, technology, and change management or health policy, ethics, and technology. The programmes at the executive and postgraduate levels should attract professionals who are already pursuing a career in, for example, clinical practice or digital technology.

Digital transformation is critically dependent not only on the increasingly widespread presence of digital tools and solutions in the health sector, but also on whether their presence results in the development of new forms of cooperation and models for how health services are provided. The new ways of working, however, might not fit within the existing legal, financial, or organizational frameworks, which need to be adapted such that the health systems can quickly start using novel solutions.

New digitally enabled health services, for example, need to be adequately recognised in provider payment systems. Similarly, if digital technology augments health workers' tasks and roles, regulations need to timely allow for expanding or reassigning these tasks and roles. The implementation of digital technologies by health care organizations needs to be planned, as, in most cases, it takes a considerable amount of time of frontline health workers, which must be accounted for and allowed for.

Including the digital future in health workforce planning

Workforce planning in the health sector is particularly important, given the time and cost involved in training the main categories of health professionals. Health workforce planning should not only guide policy decisions on entry into health education programmes, but also assess the workforce implications of possible reorganizations in health service delivery, as driven by the adoption of digital innovations, among other factors. Hence a successful digital transformation also requires that health workforce planning takes into account the future digitally enabled care models.

CHAPTER 3

PUBLIC HEALTH PROFESSIONALS' ROLE IN THE DEVELOPMENT OF DIGITAL HEALTH COMPETENCIES

CONTENTS

The digitalization of health care has changed healthcare professionals' roles and responsibilities (WHO, 2020, Odendaal et al. 2020). Rapidly changing technologies and new modes of digital communication have increased the frequency at which healthcare professionals (HCPs) need to update their skillset to provide patient-centric care, for example service accessibility, care quality, individualized care and patient participation (Ahonen et al., 2015; Mattson, 2016). Additionally, changes in the professional role may require adjustment and new competences as the power balance between HCPs and patients shifts towards patients being more informed of medical and health- related issues (Borell, 2016; Nazeha et al., 2020). Therefore, HCPs need to develop their competences to match evolving patient needs, or risk being able to advance need-based patient-centric care (Baldwin et al., 2016). In addition to technical competence in using digital systems (European Commission, 2016), HCPs also need to be able to critically evaluate how digitalization has an impact on the provision of ethical patient care (Lupton, 2017) and understand how to best use digital solutions at work (Borell, 2016)

Digital health is nowadays fundamental for physicians and other healthcare workers. Despite the improvement of Information and communications technology, public health professionals are not always equipped with suitable digital health competencies. Moreover, given the recent global health emergencies, public health professionals are waking up to their limitations in this regard.

Contemporary healthcare has very tight relations with digital technology: from clinical data storage and data analysis to communication procedures, medical doctors need to interact more with digital devices every day. Digital health represents the bridge between digital technology, healthcare and society able to enhance healthcare delivery effectiveness (Chen et al., 2019) and make medicine more personalized and precise (Bhavnani et al., 2016).

Significant work has been conducted by Gray et al. to identify the educational needs of health professionals necessary for a digitally-capable workforce (Gray et al., 2014). A key factor limiting the digital health readiness of current and future health professionals is the lack of coordinated, formal education in the use of digital technologies in health (Gray et al., 2014).

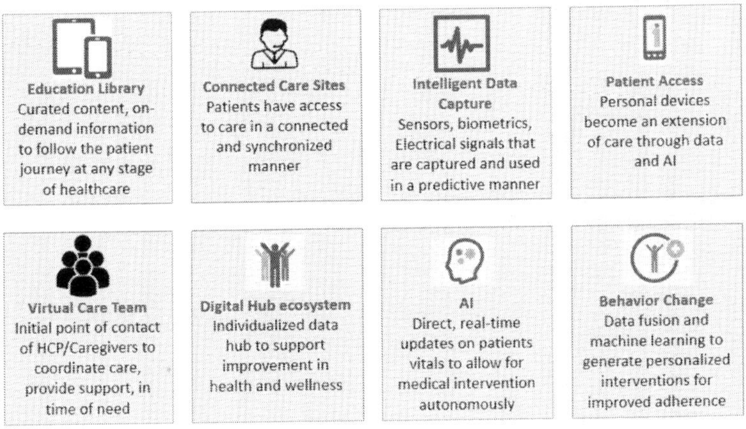

Figure 32. Building healthcare for the future.

Source: vsoftconsulting, 2022

The health practice context has become vastly more complex, mirroring changes in patients, the health system, and medical science, making it increasingly challenging for clinicians to safely and efficiently navigate health care (Obermayer at al., 2017). As digital health becomes more widespread, so does the requirement for health professionals to be well versed in navigating and using such technologies (Gray et al., 2016). Digital health education, thus, needs to be coordinated to explain and explore digital health in both current and future health care contexts, and to incorporate clear specifications as to the digital health capabilities expected of the current and future health care workforce (Gray et al., 2014).

Research into, and the development of, coordinated approaches to digital health curriculum design and implementation are necessary to effectively integrate digital health capabilities among health graduates and to support the health care workforce in using digital health technologies (Gray et al., 2016). Consequently, specific digital health education is required, even if students report to be competent and confident in using technology (Lam et al., 2016). Such skills must not be equated with technology proficiency, and most certainly not with information fluency. Information literacy is defined in essence as "the ability to access, evaluate, and use information from a variety of sources" (Doyle et al., 1990) and has become a critical skill for the present generation of students in various health-related fields (Hancock et al., 1993; Duggan 2013). For this to be achieved, a systematic approach to curriculum design and collaborative efforts from stakeholders are needed (Gray et al., 2014; Clark et al., 2009).

Although the tertiary education of health professionals is traditionally framed around a set of specific competency standards decreed by professional associations that allow measurable behaviors to be observed and assessed (O'Connell et al., 2014), competency frameworks are most beneficial when the skills and practice are consistent across contexts, for example, in the assessment of a specific injury or illness (Phelps et al., 2005). eHealth practice, on the other hand, might look different in different contexts. For example, effective integration of mobile technologies in one context might involve using mobile devices to enhance the measurement and assessment of injury. In another context, clinicians could be using apps to remotely prescribe exercises and monitor patients' physical activity. The fluidity in how eHealth skills are demonstrated across different contexts and the speed with which eHealth technologies evolve both clash with the rigidity and speed at which competencies and educational frameworks can be developed. As such, this suggests that competency standards may not be the most appropriate framing of eHealth skills and education (O'Connell et al., 2014; Phelps et al., 2005).

Investing in current and future workforce member skills will be critical for the digital transformation across all healthcare sectors: The question is how to prepare the wide range of healthcare workers, from digital natives to industry veterans, with the digital literacy capacities needed to follow through with large-scale goals.

Information and communications technologies can improve the quality and delivery of health care services around the world—particularly in low- and middle-income countries that face staffing and other physical resource constraints.

With the growing use of digital technology in health care, the roles and responsibilities of the health workforce are transforming in an unprecedented manner, intensifying the need for capacity building and continuous professional development. For example, a recent review commissioned by the United Kingdom Secretary of State for Health and Social Care (ie, the Topol Review) reported that within the next two decades, the majority of jobs in the National Health Service (NHS) will have a digital component (Topol Review, 2019). Second, the importance and potential of remote care has been brought to light recently with the COVID-19 pandemic. Virtual consultation devices and electronic systems are indispensable tools used to diagnose and treat patients with potential COVID-19 infections as well as all other infections (Government of the Republic of Korea, 2020; Mian and Khan, 2020). Third, even though the current and next generation of practitioners may be seen as "digital natives" (Aungst and Patel, 2020), surveys of health care workers show that they would appreciate more training on digital technology (Stanford Medicine, 2020; European Medical Students' Association Europe, 2019). Finally, improving digital literacy capabilities could lead to better adoption and implementation of digital services and technologies in health care settings (Royal College of Nursing, 2017). Similarly, poor digital health literacy was found to be the most common barrier to the digital transformation of health care (Schreiweis et al., 2019), and thus, the adoption of health technologies has been gradual in countries such as the United States (Adler-Milstein at al., 2014), Europe (Schreiweis et al., 2019), and Australia (National E-Health Transition Authority , 2016). For the above-mentioned reasons, there is an increasing number of medical schools introducing digital health training into their curricula (Aungst and Patel, 2020; Mesko et al., 2015; Pathipati et al., 2016)).

Such training programs should be guided by a clear framework of digital health competencies suited for different health care worker groups, settings, contexts, seniority, and role. Although there is an increasing number of individual digital health competency frameworks and reviews focusing on a specific health care worker role or setting (Chang et al., 2011; Curran, 2003; Strudwick et al., 2019; Gonçalves et al., 2012), there is a need for consolidation, analysis, and a comprehensive overview of existing frameworks for all health care worker groups. This includes frameworks that are specific for and those that are relevant across different health professions, roles, or settings. Such an overview is important to inform increasingly interdisciplinary teams working in medicine and health care and corresponding future training initiatives, policy development, and research.

Investing in current and future workforce member skills will be critical for the digital transformation across all healthcare sectors: The question is how to prepare the wide range of healthcare workers, from digital natives to industry veterans, with the digital literacy capacities needed to follow through with large-scale goals.

Doctors are particularly critical in the process of implementing digital health in the healthcare sector. Given the role of doctors in guiding patient treatment, digital health is unlikely to be routinely implemented unless they are engaged in its use. For this to happen, digital health must become an integrated part of medical education. While there have been calls for its inclusion into medical curricula, digital health is not routinely included in medical education - although digital health courses prior to and during medical school do exist (Chandrasheka, 2019; Khurana, 2020; Rosenman and Swanson, 2020; Aungst and Patel, 2020). In order for a systematic integration to occur, consensus regarding the topics to include, as well as those not to include, in such a curriculum need to be established.

Some medical schools have implemented digital health courses, although their integration thus far has been heterogenous. In a recent scoping review of digital health courses in medical schools, the authors found that the majority of courses were elective and mainly focused on medical informatics (Tudor et al, 2021). They are thus not routinely integrated into the curriculum and tend to focus on narrow topics within digital health. In Germany, following the implementation of a 3-week curricular module on digital health at a medical school, the module was well-received by both faculty and students, both of which highlighted the importance of digital health for clinical care and its underrepresentation in the curriculum (Poncette et al., 2020). From an implementation perspective, however, there are justifiable concerns regarding the already packed medical curriculum, with fears of information overload (Smith, 2010; Wartman and Combs, 2019). Identifying and removing outdated topics, which may follow directly from the automatization of certain clinical functions as digital health solutions become more commonplace, is therefore equally important in developing an optimal medical curriculum (McCoy et al., 2020).

HEALTHCARE PROFESSIONALS' PERCEPTIONS OF DIGITAL HEALTH COMPETENCE

Many health workers already use some digital tools and solutions in their daytoday work and perceive the benefits that they bring to them and to patients. However, many also question the value digital technologies produce in health care or complain about technology getting in the way of their work. Moreover, health workers often report not having opportunities for the up-skilling required to put technology to full use or that the legal and organizational aspects of work – designed in the pre digital era – are not adequately reformed to enable the technology to add value. The workers and patients also demand appropriate safeguards against potential undesired effects of the use of digital tools, including the possible lack of transparency or threats to data privacy.

In order to enable a successful digital transformation of health systems and overcome barriers governments need to provide the necessary political leadership and implement a range of policy actions to support three main objectives:

- build trust in the benefits of digital transformation among health workers and patients while minimizing any risks, which requires guaranteeing proper assessment of technology;
- advance the expertise and skills needed for the safe and effective use of digital health technologies;
- adapt the institutional environment – i.e. the legal, financial, and organizational frameworks – to enable the full potential of the technologies.

Most doctors and dentists who are asked to provide clinical leadership in eHealth within their organizations are unlikely to have undergone any formal training in informatics and will continue to work as practicing clinicians in their own specialties. In the majority of cases the eHealth role is seen as a secondary area of specialist interest, or some clinicians may be provided with dedicated time to undertake this role as part of their job plan. In a small number of cases, such as those in regional or national leadership roles, eHealth will be the primary focus of work for the medical or dental practitioner.

Healthcare professionals need to adjust to the digital era to provide quality and ethical care. Previous research has rarely adopted a healthcare professional's standpoint to describe their perceptions of digital health competence, even though their perspective in how new care practices are designed and implemented is vital.

The digitalization of health care has changed healthcare professionals' roles and responsibilities (WHO, 2020, Odendaal et al. 2020). Rapidly changing technologies and new modes of digital communication have increased the frequency at which healthcare professionals need to update their skillset to provide patient-centric care, for example service accessibility, care quality, individualized care and patient participation (Ahonen et al., 2015; Mattson, 2016). Additionally, changes in the professional role may require adjustment and new competences as the power balance between HCPs and patients shifts towards patients being more informed of medical and health-related issues (Borell, 2016; Nazeha et al., 2020). Therefore, healthcare professionals need to develop their competences to match evolving patient needs, or risk being able to advance need-based patient-centric care (Baldwin et al., 2016). In addition to technical competence in using digital systems (European Commission, 2016), HCPs also need to be able to critically evaluate how digitalization has an impact on the provision of ethical patient care (Lupton, 2017) and understand how to best use digital solutions at work (Borell, 2016).

HCPs include nurses and licenced allied health professionals (e.g. occupational therapists, physiotherapists and paramedics) who work in the healthcare field and aspire to improve and support health outside the fields of nursing and medicine (WHO, 2016, Cambridge Dictionary, 2020, UAS Act 2014/932). To ensure service efficiency in health care, HCPs need to have up-to-date competence in using digital health in their work. Simultaneously, critical digital health studies have reminded that concerns such as the digital divide causing inequalities, issues with patient integrity and safety, and the work environment of HCPs need to be addressed and resolved from the perspective of competence in digital health (Erlingsdóttir & Sandberg, 2016; Lupton, 2014). Patients are generally accepting of digital health solutions (Wass et al., 2017; Zanaboni & Fagerlund, 2020), while digital health services have been shown to positively affect various aspects of patient well-being, for example adherence to medication (Jeminiwa et al., 2019) and healthy behaviors (Posadzki et al., 2016).

Healthcare professionals' perceptions of digital health competence focus on the ability to provide patient-centric care by evaluating the need and possibilities for using digital health services jointly with more traditional methods.

Training and educating health care workers to be digitally competent is important for several reasons. First, with the growing use of digital technology in health care, the roles and responsibilities of the health workforce are transforming in an unprecedented manner, intensifying the need for capacity building and continuous professional development. For example, a recent review commissioned by the United Kingdom Secretary of State for Health and Social Care (ie, the Topol Review) reported that within the next two decades, the majority of jobs in the National Health Service (NHS) will have a digital component [9]. Second, the importance and potential of remote care has been brought to light recently with the COVID-19 pandemic. Virtual consultation devices and electronic systems are indispensable tools used to diagnose and treat patients with potential COVID-19 infections as well as all other infections (Government of the Republic of Korea, 2020; Mian and Khan, 2020). Third, even though the current and next generation of practitioners may be seen as "digital natives" (Aungst and Patel, 2020), surveys of health care workers show that they would appreciate more training on digital technology (Stanford Medicine, 2020; European Medical Students' Association Europe, 2019). Finally, improving digital literacy capabilities could lead to better adoption and implementation of digital services and technologies in health care settings (Royal College of Nursing, 2017). Similarly, poor digital health literacy was found to be the most common barrier to the digital transformation of health care (Schreiweis et al., 2019), and thus, the adoption of health technologies has been gradual in countries such as the United States (Adler at al., 2014), Europe (Schreiweis et al., 2019), and Australia (National E-Health Transition Authority, 2016). For the above-mentioned reasons, there is an increasing number of medical schools introducing digital health training into their curricula (Aungst and Patel, 2020; Mesko et al., 2020; Pathipati et al., 2016).

Such training programs should be guided by a clear framework of digital health competencies suited for different health care worker groups, settings, contexts, seniority, and role.

CHAPTER 4

DEVELOPMENT OF DIGITAL HEALTH COMPETENCIES

CONTENTS

On average today, the health systems consume a tenth of the respective national incomes, with the growth of health expenditure outpacing economic growth for most of the past half century (Lorenzoni et al., 2019[1]) – a trend that is likely to persist in the future, especially considering the impact of the current COVID19 pandemic. More efficient spending, whilst still improving the access to and the quality of health services, is a key policy challenge.

In this context, digital transformation offers unique opportunities to strengthen health systems and meet the challenges of responding to the changing health needs of the public and health workforce shortages. Many sectors in the economy have already transformed their business models for the digital era, resulting in better products and services, more efficient processes, as well as lower prices and easier access to goods and services for consumers (OECD, 2019). In the health sector, the potential benefits of digital technologies and digitally driven process innovation are abundant. Ensuring access to the right information by the right people at the right time can improve safety, effectiveness, and efficiency of care. Digitally enhanced health services can improve access and help move away from reactive towards proactive approaches to preserving health. Health workers could be relieved from time consuming routine tasks and interact better with patients

Digital health will be valued and adopted if it:

- is accessible and supports equitable and universal access to quality health services
- enhances the efficiency and sustainability of health systems in delivering quality, affordable and equitable care
- strengthens and scales up health promotion, disease prevention, diagnosis, management, rehabilitation and palliative care including before, during and after an epidemic or pandemic, in a system that respects the privacy and security of patient health information.

The vision further seeks to enhance research and development, innovation and collaboration across sectors. It recognizes that digital health can radically change health outcomes if it is supported by sufficient investment in governance, institutional and workforce capacity to enable the changes in digital systems and data use training, planning, and management that are required as health systems and services are increasingly digitized. With this essential investment in people and processes, in line with national strategies that lay out a vision for the digitalization of the health sector, digital health can improve the efficiency and cost-effectiveness of care, allowing for new business models in the delivery of services. Drawing on experiences in developing countries, digital health thought leaders have developed a framework of 12 common digital health competencies to develop for reproductive, maternal, newborn and child health (RMNCH) as shown on the table below. These include using technology for behavior change communication, data collection and provider training, and highlight a range of possibilities that practitioners may consider for their programs and context.

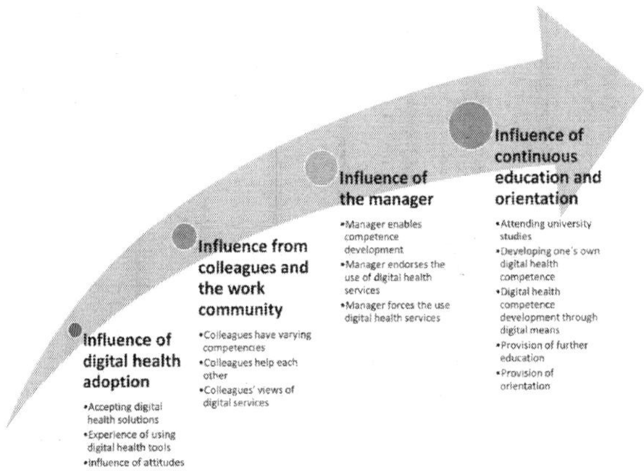

Figure 33. Digital Health Competence Development.

Source: Jarva et al., 2022

Table 3. Identified digital health competencies for reproductive, maternal, newborn and child health

1. Client education and behavior change communication (BCC)	7. Provider-to-provider communication ser groups, consultation
2. Sensors and point-of-care diagnostics	8. Provider work planning and scheduling
3. Registries/vital events tracking	9. Provider training and education
4. Data collection and reporting	10. Human resource management
5. Electronic health records	11. Supply chain management
6. Electronic decision support Information, protocols, algorithms, checklists	12. Financial transactions and incentives
Credit: Labrique AB, Vasudevan L, Kochi E, Fabricant R, & Mehl G.	

Practitioners also have to answer other questions as they plan for mHealth, including: What human resources are needed to support such a project? Do we build a tool in-house or engage the services of a partner organization? How much will a digital health system cost to implement and manage? How will we implement the project? How will we measure its success?

These questions can help practitioners objectively evaluate the need and value of digital health for their program, rather than adopting a digital health intervention because it sounds appealing, because others have done so or because donors wish to fund it.

This process also highlights the nuances of implementing and managing a digital health program, reveals key human-resource, financial and other considerations, and uncovers potential challenges to be addressed. A variety of toolkits have been designed to guide practitioners as they plan for mHealth and other digital health programs. For example, a toolkit from the World Health Organization and PATH lays out an eight-step process that can help practitioners develop their program along with planning tools for each step.

Toolkits such as these can help practitioners conceptualize their digital health programs, but even the best-laid plans often go awry once the work of design and implementation actually begins. How then do you get from an mHealth plan to the actual practice of it? Below, we propose a 10 step plan for the development of digital competencies.

Table 4. 10 Step Plan for the Development of Digital Health Competencies

Step	**Points to be considered**
1. Define Outcomes	How will a better information system benefit you? How should you define the scope? How will you measure success?
2. Form a Team	What skills and roles are required to bring your project to a satisfying outcome?
3. Define what your System needs to do	How can you define your requirements for the system?
4. Find the right Solution	Should you buy or build your system? Do you select an open-source or proprietary system? How do you evaluate different systems and select the best one?

<table>
<tr><td>5. Select the right Vendors</td><td>How do you make sure you select the best providers of technical services?</td></tr>
<tr><td colspan="2">6. Estimate Implementation and Operating Costs
How much will your project cost to pilot, scale and maintain?</td></tr>
<tr><td>7. Create an Implementation Plan</td><td>How long will it take to develop, pilot and scale up?</td></tr>
<tr><td>8. Understand and Manage Project risks</td><td>What can go wrong and how can you plan for that?</td></tr>
<tr><td>9. Evaluate the outcomes</td><td>Have the targeted outcomes been achieved in a measurable scale?</td></tr>
<tr><td>10. Adjust as required</td><td>What changes need to be made to the system/program in order to meet or improve defined outcomes?</td></tr>
</table>

Successful implementation requires a skilled and trained workforce to support the use and maintenance of newly developed digital health tools. Although public health programs are well versed in delivering training, digital health training can pose unique challenges. Users differ in their digital literacy or baseline knowledge of technology and may have varying learning curves, irrespective of their level of education and area of expertise. Building capacity and planning for continued end-user training after implementation is a non-negotiable investment of resources for the success of digital health competency.

Another crucial aspect is management and supervision of the tool or program. Implementation may imply finality, but is in fact the completion of only one iteration of the entire process. Being open to continuous iteration with users even after implementation is crucial for the tool to evolve into a more enhanced and impactful solution over time.

FRAMEWORK COMPONENTS FOR REGULATING DIGITAL HEALTH COMPETENCY PROGRAMS

Three capabilities—the Regulatory Development Kit (RDK), FDA Pre-Cert, and the Multi- Stakeholder Real World Data Capability—comprise the core components of the proposed framework for establishing a regulated digital health competency program.

Regulatory Development Kit

While SaMD products are not new, there are many new players in the digital health competency space, including tech giants and start- ups that see opportunities to contribute their talents and expertise to digital health but may be unfamiliar with FDA regulatory processes. However, new players aren't the only ones who may require regulatory assistance. Given the speed with which the FDA is evolving to better regulate iterative devices all digital health competency developers likely could benefit from timely information on FDA requirements and guidance on how to interact with the agency to get their products to market. An important step forward is to make the regulatory process easier for digital health competency developers to understand and navigate.

Enter the Regulatory Development Kit (RDK). The FDA has been considering creating a RDK to help digital health technology developers easily understand and meet the agency's regulatory requirements. As such, it could be

useful to outfit the RDK with a module that functions similar to a software program that guides individuals through a step-by-step process to complete their federal and state income tax forms—in this case, the RDK could guide users through the regulatory process. The RDK could contain tools to clarify requirements and expectations at each stage of the process; provide templates to accelerate development of required documentation; and supply answers to frequently asked questions about data standardization, security requirements, and legal and clinical information. The RDK also could contain an expert-monitored wiki for users to share leading practices. In short, the RDK could provide the healthcare industry with a simple, user-friendly guide to the digital health competency regulatory process, thus encouraging future product innovation and proliferation.

FDA Pre-Cert

The FDA has limited resources with which to evaluate new digital health competency before they are introduced into the market. According to Bakul Patel, FDA Associate Director for Digital Heath, the volume of FDA premarket approval applications for digital health competency has the potential to increase exponentially as technology advances spawn development of more software-based health care solutions. A risk-based approach to regulatory review could allow the FDA to accelerate review for lower-risk digital health competency and focus its attention and limited resources on reviewing SaMDs that pose greater potential risk of causing patient harm.

One proposed regulatory review option—an FDA Pre-Cert Program to facilitate expedited digital health competency approvals—is inspired by the TSA Preümodel (see sidebar). The FDA Pre-Cert Program would be a risk-based, expedited, and predictable approval process for organizations that demonstrate a commitment to a culture of quality and organizational excellence (CQOE). Entry into this new pathway would be contingent on the digital health competency developer providing access to key pieces of pre- and post-market information to provide continued confidence in the product's safety, efficacy, and performance. Two factors could be used to determine the pre- and post-market requirements for each digital health competency review:

(1) the digital health competency organization's standing in the FDA Pre-Cert Program; and

(2) the risk categorization of the digital health competency being evaluated.

Organizations that demonstrate a commitment to organizational excellence could expect to spend relatively less (or no) time in pre-market review than their non-Pre-Cert peers with similarly risky products; however, higher-risk products may have more requirements than lower-risk ones.

Pre-Cert eligibility: Measuring an organization's commitment to excellence

FDA Pre-Cert eligibility would be determined based on a company's ability to demonstrate a culture of quality and organizational excellence (CQOE). The proposed CQOE framework comprises two core components, organizational perspectives and excellence outcomes.

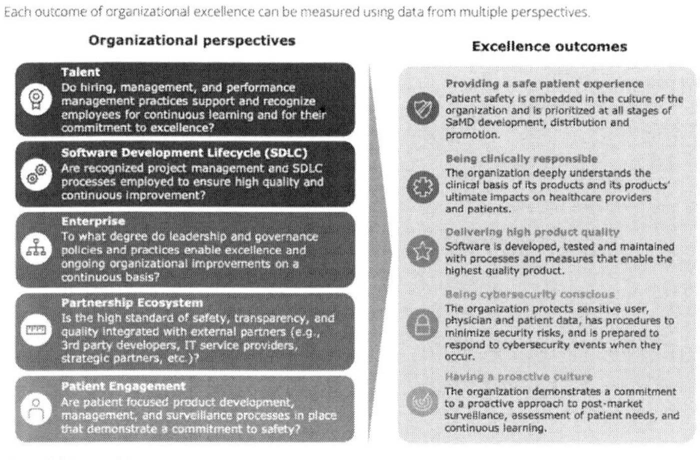

Figure 34. Culture of Quality and Organizational Excellence (CQOE) framework.

Source: Deloitte Analysis, 2022

- Organizational perspectives are areas that the FDA could evaluate to determine a SaMD organization's quality and commitment to excellence. Our framework proposes the organizational perspectives of talent, software development life cycle (SDLC), enterprise, partnership ecosystem, and patient engagement. The perspectives, which link to the FDA's proposed excellence outcomes (described below), would be self-reported and measured through a standard set of (yet-to-be-determined) KPIs and measures; quantified through an overall aggregate CQOE score; and displayed via an organizational excellence scorecard, with Bronze, Silver, and Gold levels reflecting a company's overall commitment to quality. The organizational perspectives would indicate the likelihood of a company's ability to create devices that meet the FDA's standards for excellence.
- Excellence outcomes are results that show a SaMD organization's products meet the FDA's standards for excellence and quality. These excellence outcomes include providing a safe patient experience, being clinically responsible, delivering high-quality products, being conscious of cybersecurity, and having a proactive culture

Because the data used to assess organizational perspectives would be self-reported, it raises the risk of a company submitting inaccurate or falsified information to gain Pre-Cert status. To address this situation, the FDA could incorporate automated audit techniques using advanced audit and AI methods to identify and prevent fraud.

ONGOING ASSESSMENT OF PRODUCT SAFETY AND EFFECTIVENESS

Whether the organization is established or new, large or small, all market entrants will have the opportunity to apply and qualify for Pre-Cert. Even organizations that already have SaMD products in the market could be evaluated on the safety and effectiveness of those products and be eligible for Pre-Cert. The FDA could continuously track these measures through the Real World Data Capability and incorporate the results dynamically into the CQOE score and respective Pre-Cert level. The FDA also could monitor products through publicly available data on software bugs and error reports, customer feedback, software updates, app store information, social media, and GitHub.

CQOE scores and corresponding Pre-Cert levels wouldn't be static: they could go up or down based on performance and effectiveness data gathered through the RWDC, app store reviews and other data already being gathered on the device. If a CQOE score were to fall below a defined Pre-Cert threshold (e.g., moving from Pre-Cert Gold to Silver), the organization may lose certain Pre-Cert benefits, such as expedited reviews for less-risky SaMD products, or it may no longer be eligible for FDA Pre-Cert status until it is able to demonstrate a commitment to excellence through a new Pre-Cert assessment and resolution of any product issues.

RISK CATEGORIZATION

An important consideration for an FDA Pre-Cert and expedited review pathway is evaluating the level of risk posed by a SaMD. One potential model is the SaMD Risk Categorization Framework developed and published by the International Medical Device Regulators Forum (IMDRF). While different from existing medical device classification (e.g., Class 1, 2, 3), it plays a similar function in enabling the FDA to risk-stratify submissions and focus resources on products that pose the greatest risk to patient safety.

Higher-risk devices (Category IV) may require a thorough clinical evaluation through clinical trials or retrospective analysis of existing clinical information to ensure safety, effectiveness, and performance. However, even Category IV devices could be eligible for FDA Pre-Cert expedited review, depending on specific product attributes, such

as the clinical efficacy and safety evidence provided to support approval, as well as a company's Pre-Cert level and other product attributes that can potentially pose a safety risk to patients. For example, a company with the highest CQOE score and Pre-Cert level (e.g., Gold) might be able to submit a Category IV device within the same timeframe and with the same burden of requirements as a Category III device with a less favorable CQOE score and Pre-Cert level (e.g., Silver).

Low-risk devices (Category I) could skip the review altogether, per FDA guidance,29 and Category II devices may similarly be eligible to skip review or undergo an expedited review process wherein the manufacturer could simply submit an application and go straight to market without waiting for approval but with a commitment to share RWD to enable FDA to monitor all SaMD products post-market. A combination of the organization's Pre-Cert standing and the device's individual risk categorization would determine the amount of premarket review required for each SaMD. An organization's Pre-Cert standing would be dynamic and change over time based on real world post-market performance of products and audits of the organizational excellence metrics and KPIs provided by the organization.

BARRIERS TO ADOPTION OF DIGITAL HEALTH IN DEVELOPING COUNTRIES

High Implementation and Maintenance Costs

The cost of EHR implementation is one of the most frequently identified factors that limit EHR adoption. Studies have shown that low adoption of EHR in sub-Saharan Africa can be linked to high costs of implementation and maintenance due to hardware, software, training, and support costs (Akanbi et al., 2012; Awokola et al., 2012). Many hospitals and physicians in sub-Saharan African countries were mainly concerned about the large capital outlay (Fraser et al., 2005; Williams and Boren, 2008; Pantuvo et al., 2011; Akanbi et al., 2012; Awokola et al., 2012) associated with hardware, software, and installation; broadband connection costs; the cost of accessories such as scanners, printers, paper, and ink; and recurring expenses for system maintenance. Furthermore, Akanbi *et al.* stated that lack of robust/poor infrastructure in developing nations also increased both the costs of setting up EHR and costs of maintenance (Williams and Bore, 2008; Akanbi et al., 2012). Awokola *et al.* pointed out that the software used in health-care establishments is very expensive and that a basic EHR costs about $32,000 excluding technical support and ongoing maintenance (Awokola et al., 2012). As a result of high costs of EHR procurement, many hospitals, though beneficial in a number of other ways, did not see EHR implementation as a priority (Awokola et al., 2012).

Limited Computer Skills

Low computer literacy level is another variable that clearly emerged from the articles reviewed as one of the potent factors that limit the wider adoption of EHR in sub-Saharan African countries. Physicians reported a series of skill-related factors that they believe would make it difficult to use an EHR. These included lack of typing proficiency, low/no understanding of how to use a computer, lack of understanding of how to use the EHR system, and inability to type while talking with patients (Cline, 2013; Awokola et al., 2011; Ameh et al., 2008). The study conducted on computer and internet use by doctors in one of the sub-Saharan African countries showed that the overall proficiency of the respondents in computer based competencies was below average. Only 32 (26.7%) were sufficiently familiar with computer tools to perform advanced tasks (Awokola et al., 2011). The researchers stated further that the Appalachian Regional Informatics Consortium Survey of 2005 in Ohio, United States, showed that 91.4% of doctors could use an EHR. In the Canadian Medical Association physician resource survey of 2000, 84% of doctors showed computer use proficiency. Similarly, higher values were seen in a study of student doctors in Malaysia in 2002, where 94.4% of the subjects could use a computer well (Awokola et al., 2011). As a result of low-level computer literacy in the sub-Saharan African countries, many physicians and other key end users are not eager/willing to adopt an EHR and ultimately low EHR adoption in the region.

Poor Electricity Supply and Lack of Constant Internet Connectivity

Lack of constant supply of electricity has also been identified by many researchers as a major barrier to a successful wider implementation and adoption of EHR in this region (Pantuvo et al., 2011; Williams and Boren,

2008; Oluoch et al., 2012; Awokola et al., 2012). For instance, Awokola *et al.*, reported that for many months, they could not use the EHR consistently because of the constant power outage. In addition, Pantuvo *et al.* stated that many hospitals in this region do not have access to constant electricity supply (Pantuvo et al., 2011). In fact, many hospitals depend mainly on the alternative power supply commonly called "generator" for their operations. Due to the infrastructure issues all through the nation and absence of guaranteed internet connection or even uncertain continuous power supply (Chaplin et al., 2015; Pantuvo et al., 2011; Williams and Boren, 2008) a wider implementation of EHR in some sub-Saharan nations may not be conceivable. Furthermore, the study conducted on the use of health information and communication technologies by health workers in seven state hospitals and a private hospital in the North Eastern Zone, Ogun State, Nigeria, reported that only one of the hospitals examined was connected to the internet, and none of them had a website (Ajiboye et al., 2014). Jimoh *et al.* noted that the internet penetration was very low. For instance, the internet penetration of <16% and average broadband download speed of 1.38 mbps (compared with 10.1 mbps the United States (Jimoh et al., 2012). Overall, poor electricity supply and lack of constant internet connectivity have been reported as strong barriers to EHR adoption in this region.

Lack of Prioritization of EHR

Studies have shown that most developing countries face many challenges ranging from disease epidemics to civil wars to disasters so EHR implementation may seem outside the priority agenda in this region (Williams and Bore, 2008; Blaya et al., 2010). Akanbi *et al.* revealed that most EHRs in this region were sustained by funding from foreign partnerships, thereby raising the question about the sustainability of these systems by the domestic institutions. Many countries in sub-Saharan Africa did not have a specific policy in place on EHR adoption and no financial incentives for adoption (Williams and Bore, 2008; Blaya et al., 2010; Hillestad et al., 2005; Akanbi et al., 2012).

FACTORS FACILITATING THE ADOPTION OF DIGITAL HEALTH IN DEVELOPING COUNTRIES

Implementation Planning

Comprehensive planning before implementation was frequently cited in literature. Planning steps included setting realistic goals and expectations, involving EHR users early in the planning process, determining how current workflows will be redefined with EHRs, system selection, staged implementation processes, and learning from facilities that have implemented EHR systems (Pantuvo et al., 2011; Williams and Boren, 2008; Fraser and Playa, 2010).

Training and Education

Training of EHR users was also reported in studies to be an effective strategy for getting end users' acceptance. Training should be both initial and ongoing (Pantuvo et al., 2011; Williams and Boren, 2008; Fraser and Playa, 2010). Physicians and other EHR end users have to set time aside to study how the system is operated and how their workflow should be redesigned to allow for an efficient use of the system. Training, however, should commence with the most interested EHR users, the so-called local champions who will subsequently be used to motivate the others and developed to "super users" to handle most basic hardware and software problems locally (Fraser and Blaya, 2010). Equally, incorporation of health informatics into the school curriculum by the academic health institutions that train medical doctors, pharmacist, nurses, laboratory scientists, and other health workers were frequently mentioned by researchers (Pantuvo et al., 2011; Castelnuovo et al., 2012).

Financial Supports

In addition, literature supports the notion that financial assistance from the government to cover implementation costs. This can be in the form of grants or one-time payments for infrastructure and hardware costs, reimbursement incentives. Many researchers pointed out that some form of government incentives would be required to see substantial adoption and meaningful use of EHR in sub-Saharan African countries (Pantuovo et al., 2011; Blaya et al., 2010).

Appropriate EHR System Selection

Studies have shown that while it is true that the cost of implementation of an EHR can be prohibitive for most developing countries, the use of low-cost technologies has been demonstrated to be sustainable in many such countries (Fraser at al., 2005; Pantuovo et al., 2011; Blaya et al., 2010; Kamadjeu et al., 2005; Rotich et al., 2003). "The functionality of EHR systems varies across multiple settings. To be most useful, a functional model of an EHR system must reflect a balance between what is desirable and what can feasibly be implemented immediately or within a short time frame." (Institute of Medicine, 2003).

Phased Implementation

Another strategy that facilitates EHR adoption in sub-Saharan Africa is the embracing of phased implementation. According to Pantuvo et al., a phased implementation involves implementing one unit at a time. The author stated that "a phased implementation is preferred for resource-constrained areas where the resources to tackle all the issues that implementation will raise are not readily available. This gives room to manage changes in small units and transfer lessons learned to other units." (Pantuovo et al., 2011).

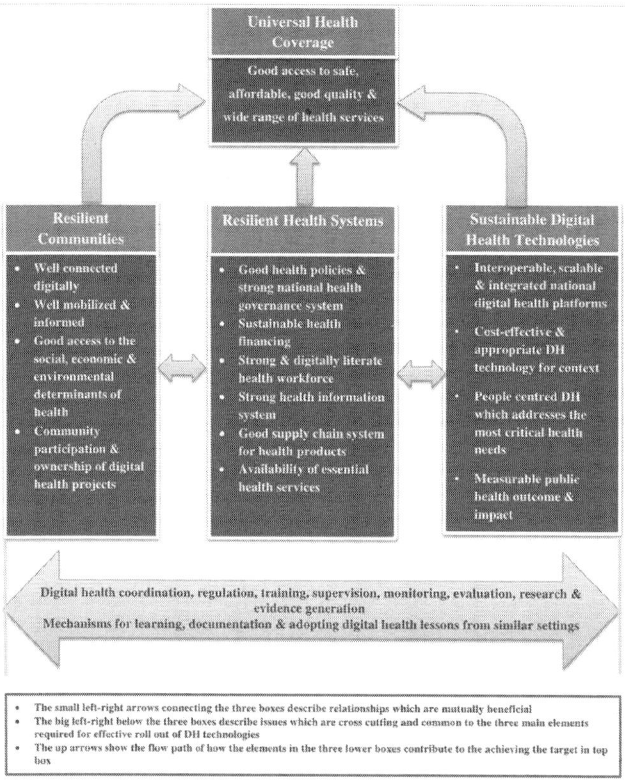

Figure 35. Proposed conceptual framework for rapid and effective scale up of digital health technologies in Africa.

Source: Olu et al., 2019

INCREASING DIGITAL SKILLS AMONG HEALTHCARE PROFESSIONALS

Health care is catching up digitally compared to other industries. From the perspective of the doctor, nurse, or administrative staff, this means learning many new IT system functionalities quickly. On top of that, you have to add ongoing changes in the software resulting from new administrative regulations.

What's more, medical staff often work in different medical facilities with different software. Workers have different initial digital skills. Technology itself is also changing: organizations are moving to cloud solutions; mobile devices are replacing desktop computers; documentation is increasingly recorded by voice; clinical decision support systems are imposing new working procedures; system updates require new knowledge.

Whether healthcare workers can adapt to the rapidly changing environment depends on a well-planned programme of continuous competence development. This consists of six pillars:

- Defining the measurable skill rates
- Communication of objectives and a timetable for digitalization
- Planning of training adapted to different groups
- Systematic improvement of digital competences
- Assessing digital skills
- … and improving them.

How to measure skills

The first point may be crucial. At this stage, it is necessary to separate soft skills, such as the ease of using a computer, the speed of entering data into the system, or the ability to facilitate one's own work by appropriate settings of IT system options. These elements should be subject to observation and be part of systematic competence improvement but are not baseline. Measuring the speed of entering patient data into the system would probably be the worst idea, leading only to harmful psychological pressure.

The elements that determine vital indicators should be prioritized: patient safety, financial situation, and quality of services. Systematic reviews of the quality of the data entered, and audits can be a measure.

Managing digital transformation

A strategic element is to inform the staff why a new system is being introduced, and even better, to involve them in the change process so that they better understand the expected outcomes of innovation. Improving the coordination of treatment or the financial situation are more convincing arguments than generally formulated "digitalization."

Within the framework of "onboarding" new employees, the starting point is a questionnaire to determine the baseline skills. As a result, different user groups can be identified, and an appropriate training cycle can be tailored. Improving digital skills and, thus, innovation should become part of the organizational culture.

Training plus individual advice

The introduction of any new system functionality should be followed by know-how – training on test data, well-prepared documentation. The training must include various toolboxes, from general group workshops conducted by the software manufacturer to individual meetings or online webinars for self-learning at any time. In case of urgent questions, in order not to impede work, the employee must be able to quickly contact an expert through a chat with the IT department or a conversation with a mentor appointed on behalf of the manufacturer / IT company.

A series of training sessions on a new system is just the beginning. Every organization needs a strategy for continuous competence improvement. In large organizations, such as hospitals, it is best to appoint a leader in each department who is fluent in the IT infrastructure and, based on observation of the employees' work, makes suggestions to the management for improving competencies. This type of coach is closest to the employee and can respond to urgent questions on an ongoing basis.

Digital skills should be measured systematically – not to control/punish employees but to develop their competencies to facilitate their daily duties. Everyone will agree that the seamless operation of an IT system has a positive impact on job satisfaction. A lack of digital skills, on the other hand, can be not only frustrating but also dangerous, leading to professional burnout.

The bare minimum of skills measurement includes cyber security audits conducted by the IT department. For example, does the employee open suspicious emails and click on the links they contain? Do they log off the system during breaks?

In recent years, we have seen significant progress in the ergonomics of IT systems. Manufacturers are constantly adjusting them to the user's expectations, introducing new interfaces, making versions of systems available for convenient operation on mobile devices.

However, the value and benefits of any IT system depend primarily on the employees' knowledge of how to use it. So it is worth building a coherent strategy for improving skills. Information about IT systems, modules, new functions need to be structured, made available on-demand on the local network in various formats – from printed manuals to instructional videos so that everyone can learn at their own pace, in the way they prefer.

The responsibility for the comfort of working with the IT system is shared between the medical facility and the software provider. Therefore, purchasing software is not just a transaction but ideally involves establishing a close relationship with the supplier. For example, the IT company will benefit from suggestions made by frontline employees and will be able to incorporate them into future software versions. In turn, the organization gains influence on the shape of the system.

And finally, the essential element – continuous learning. A new tomograph or computer usually requires a one-time training session. New functions are introduced to the software on an ongoing basis. Many of them are not used at all but could significantly improve the quality of work. This also applies to some options available in the systems – their appropriate configuration can save a few seconds of data recording, which translates into dozens of minutes a day.

Infrastructure Defines the Limits of Digital Health Access and Use

Digital health, like every other digital service, relies on physical infrastructure. People, businesses, and government agencies need to have access to reliable and affordable Internet services, whether they are broadband or mobile networks. LMICs and their development partners need to address this costly and complicated issue before they can even get to the issues around the digital applications that rely on the Internet. Therefore, closing the infrastructure gap in developing countries will be critical to closing the digital health divide.

Table 5. Opportunities for Health Care Organizations to Increase Digital Inclusion through Infrastructure Initiatives

Infrastructure Investment and Jobs Act Policy Area	Opportunities for Health Care Organizations
Broadband infrastructure	Collect information on patients' broadband access to identify broadband coverage gaps and guide allocation of infrastructure-building resources Ensure that digital health tools can adapt to potential bandwidth limitations
Broadband and device affordability	Develop workflows that integrate digital-inclusion resources into existing care (e.g., screening for social determinants of health) Perform targeted outreach to patients who would benefit from broadband and device-subsidies programs (e.g., Emergency Broadband Benefit) Join existing digital-inclusion efforts (e.g., programs addressing digital divides in education) led by community organizations
Digital discrimination	Advocate for equitable broadband-deployment practices at the local, state, and national levels Collect patient data regarding digital disparities (e.g., disparities in broadband and device access) to support multimodal care options Treat digital inclusion as a social determinant of health
Digital literacy	Apply for funding with community organizations to codevelop digital-literacy programs that extend beyond the health care setting Integrate digital navigation as part of the deployment of digital health tools

Source: Rodríguez et al., 2022

Digital health is growing in relevance and scale as more and more people access the Internet—at the end of 2018, it was estimated that over half of the world's population was using the Internet (ITU, 2018). However, there is significant variation in coverage and accessibility of mobile cellular networks, especially where they are needed most: In the world's 47 least-developed countries, more than 80 percent of the population is still offline (ITU, 2019). This directly affects the ability of countries to deliver digital health programs. Not surprisingly, according to the Global Digital Health Index (which draws on the World Economic Forum's Network Readiness Index), the maturity of digital health infrastructure has a strong correlation with a country's stage of development (Mechael and Edelman, 2019). However, the Index notes that some countries are focused on addressing the gap through plans to improve infrastructure for public health facilities and offices, with Bangladesh, Jordan, and Thailand particular standouts.

ICT infrastructure (along with energy) attracts two-thirds of private infrastructure financing in LMICs, in large part due to the capital intensity of the sector and the clear commercial opportunities in providing Internet connectivity (Tyson, 2028). But this is not the case across all LMICs. This leaves gaps where national governments and development agencies have a clearer role to step in. However, development agencies have not yet deployed much capital (or attention) to improving ICT infrastructure in LMICs as part of a holistic digital development strategy. At the moment, only a small proportion of development budgets go to helping LMICs improve their ICT infrastructure. Only 1 percent of all funding provided under what are known as "Aid for Trade" programs is currently allocated to ICT solutions. Similarly, multilateral development banks are investing just 1 percent of their total investment in ICT projects (World Wide Web Foundation, 2018).

Box 16. Recommendations for the development of digital health competency frameworks

Methodology:

- Literature review, followed by consultations or Delphi study with local experts, followed by engagement with international experts

Content:

- Explore new competency areas that appeared in recent frameworks (ie, attitudes and advocacy toward the use of information technology (IT), medication management, public health)
- Update competencies based on technological innovations and adoption and emerging evidence (ie, health apps, artificial intelligence, autonomous decision-support systems)
- Include essential interprofessional competencies (ie, informatics concepts and processes, health information management, communication, ethics, legal, or regulations, and privacy and security)

Target audience or setting to include:

- Allied health professionals
- Low- and middle-income countries

Application:

- Provide case studies of integration into curricula or training programs or examples of application in practice

Development agencies need to consider the specific impact that gaps in ICT connectivity have on digital health plans and programs, and come up with plans and resources to help close them. It's unlikely private-sector financing will address all gaps in connectivity, as not all projects (such as in rural areas) will be commercially viable for private firms. National governments and development partners should work together to come up with policies and resources to help build ICT infrastructure in these areas. This could include new business models that aggregate demand among public buyers who want to reach marginalized and remote people, thus helping to facilitate the development of local markets for the provision of health care and other digital services—and providing incentives to make requisite investments. Given those countries and communities that remain disconnected also stand to benefit the most from digital technologies, improving their connectivity should be a top priority.

CHAPTER 5

WHAT THE FUTURE HOLDS

CONTENTS

In the health sector, the potential benefits of digital technologies are abundant. Ensuring access to the right information by the right people at the right time can improve safety, effectiveness, and efficiency of care. Digitally enhanced health services can improve access and help move away from reactive towards proactive approaches to preserving health. Health workers could be relieved from time consuming routine tasks and interact better with patients. Patients could become more engaged, improve self care skills, and more effectively coproduce health.

Successful digital transformation in the health sector is not a simple matter of technical change but requires a complex adaptive change in human attitudes and skills as well as in the organization of work and the related legal and financial frameworks. Digital technologies only provide the tools and cannot transform the health sector on its own but need to be put to productive use by the health workers and patients.

Many health workers already use some digital tools and solutions in their daytoday work and perceive the benefits that they bring to them and to patients. However, many also question the value digital technologies produce in health care or complain about technology getting in the way of their work. Moreover, health workers often report not having opportunities for the up-skilling required to put the technology to full use or that the legal, financial, and organizational aspects of work – designed in the pre digital era – are not adequately reformed to enable the technology to add value. The workers and patients also demand appropriate safeguards against potential undesired effects of the use of digital tools, including the possible lack of transparency or threats to data privacy. If unaddressed, these concerns are not only likely to result in additional inefficiency and waste, but also place undue burden and strain on the workers.

Over the last three decades, there has been considerable interest in the use of digital health to enhance the quality, efficiency, and safety of health care (Catwell and Sheikh, 2009; Peckham, 2016). Digital health and eHealth are often used interchangeably and broadly defined as "the use of information and communications technology in support of health and health-related fields" (WHO, 2019). An analysis of various digital health definitions revealed three distinct yet overlapping uses such as monitoring, tracking, and informing health (eg, mobile devices, mobile sensors and wearables, apps, social media); enabling health communication among various stakeholders (eg, digital health, virtual consultations); and storing, managing, and utilizing health data (eg, electronic medical records, electronic medication systems) (Shaw et al., 2017). Digital health tools have the potential to provide health care workers with a holistic view of patients' medical conditions through access to their health-related data and improved communication, regardless of distance and access (WHO, 2016). Furthermore, the use of digital technology in health care could potentially reduce turnaround times, resource use, medication errors, and adverse drug events; increase the use of preventive care; and enable greater adherence to clinical guidelines (Keasberry et al., 2017; Nanah and Bayoumi, 2020; Mohsin et al., 2019).

TRENDS DEFINING THE FUTURE OF GLOBAL DIGITAL HEALTH

Whether on the political, scientific, or cultural front, the world today is in a state of flux. Reviews from BCG, McKinsey, Deloitte, and Accenture highlight major demographic shifts, the increasing importance of technology in health, and the convergence of business and technical considerations. Digital platforms and solutions are a source of hope, inspiration, and connection.

The Digital Health team at PATH has spent the last year reviewing global analyses, listening to end users and partners in the field, and exchanging perspectives throughout the global digital health community about issues that are both driving and impacting the global health sector.

1. Globalization and localization of digital health

As political and economic power shift to rapidly growing countries, local institutions are increasingly influential in the traditional aid sector. Local governments have the capacity and resources to invest in infrastructure and take on new levels of responsibility. Local businesses and nonprofits are increasingly capable of managing technical partnerships in support of development.

What this means for global digital health:

- Traditional donors more strongly encourage local hiring and innovation.
- International organizations curate peer networks and foster global innovation hubs that allow diverse, virtual teams to innovate and diffuse innovations faster and better.
- These global networks and hubs enable the next wave of global digital health innovations.

2. Growing power of (some) end users

The GSMA forecasts mobile internet subscriptions will hit 56% by 2020. A large percentage of these users are on social media networks, which provide a direct link between end users and local and global communities, as well as a new way to exert influence on their own health and society. This growth, however, is not equitable. Women in South Asia are 38% less likely to own a mobile phone than men, and the gender gap in digital access is growing in Africa. Digital health investors and implementers should consider gender and cultural issues to help address equity gaps.

What this means for global digital health:

- Low-income populations monitor and manage their own health digitally, resulting in lower rates of noncommunicable diseases.
- Public health programs use social media platforms to share information and gather feedback.
- Women use technology to gather critical health information, make peer connections, and link directly to experts.

3. Digital data transforms health systems

A fully digitized health system connects families living in remote areas to health providers. It diversifies and expands the biodata available for computational analysis, ensuring that innovations in personalized medicine address global needs equitably. And digitization drives down costs in health system by enabling earlier identification of disease, leaner supply chains, and more efficient operations. The enormous potential value of data can be realized with fast, high-volume, real-time data processing. Cloud-based solutions allow programs to affordably manage and find value from big data.

What this means for global digital health:

- Strong cloud-based governance and regulatory frameworks address country concerns about data sovereignty.
- Countries migrate to robust cloud-based solutions and invest in local infrastructure and staff to meet the system requirements of big data.

4. Broadening to community-wide resiliency

In our connected world, a local crisis has the potential to impact the global community. Loss of homes due to climate change, increased migration, human conflict, and extreme poverty all pose risks to health, and all require interventions that extend far beyond the traditional health system. Organizations that use information and communication technology for development, including those focused on improving health outcomes, will need to broaden beyond historic aid siloes and understand how different sectors impact each other to improve the resiliency of communities in crises.

What this means for global digital health:

- Digital platforms break down programmatic barriers by bridging data divides and proving the value of connecting silos.
- Digital platforms continue to increase responsiveness to crises and accelerate recovery timelines.
- Funders support cross-sectoral solutions that holistically address individuals and community needs.

5. Merging of digital health sectors – global with local and public with private

While health equity increases throughout the world, remaining inequality has become more visible because of increased access to information and decreasing physical proximity between the healthy and unhealthy. Twenty years ago, those with the lowest life expectancies were concentrated in low-income countries. Today, in high-income cities like Seattle in the US (where PATH is headquartered), life expectancy may vary by more than 15 years, depending on the neighborhood.

What this means for global digital health:

- The global digital health sector plays a role in supporting low-income communities in wealthy countries, bringing expertise in building solutions for low-resource settings.
- As middle-income communities grow in countries like India and China, the global digital health sector works with private-sector partners that bring more sophisticated software and services.

6. More support for human-centered care

Over the coming years, longer lifespans, demographics shifts, and a growing global middle class will alter the global burden of disease and demands on health systems. Noncommunicable, chronic conditions that require ongoing management will increase. Whether bolstering mental health or managing hypertension, interventions need to be part of a holistic, interactive solution that takes individualized, lifelong approaches.

What this means for global digital health:

- Digital tools empower end users to adopt or reinforce health behaviors (rather than delivering digital solutions via health provider intermediaries).
- Public health programs efficiently monitor the health of communities to prioritize interventions.
- Interventions that have worked for wealthier populations are adapted to work in low-resource settings.

7. More support for cost-saving solutions

Lower-income countries already struggle to resource their health systems; meanwhile, new health technologies, longer-living populations and noncommunicable diseases will continue to drive up costs per patient.

What this means for global digital health:

- Digital health interventions are developed to increase affordability of preventing, treating, and monitoring population health.
- Digital information systems provide visibility into cost-containment opportunities and enable monitoring of which solutions are successful.
- New business and health insurance models are developed to achieve universal health coverage.
- Health insurance providers have sophisticated approaches to cost containment without sacrificing patient outcomes and are increasingly present as advisors, partners, and implementers in low-resource settings.

8. Growing focus on data ownership, ethics, and rights

Demand for data has never been higher. Traditional players in the sector (including PATH) want data to improve program effectiveness and get ahead of the anti-globalization sentiment that threatens global development programs. New players (e.g., an increasingly engaged private sector) need data to learn how to best add value in the sector. Yet as data grows in value, data suppliers and owners form an increasingly complex and fragmented network, each with their own motivations for data use. This network often exists outside a comprehensive regulatory environment, creating a "wild west" atmosphere for the management and use of health data.

What this means for global digital health:

- New ownership and privacy policies protect fundamental human rights.
- Data monetization drives social outcomes (rather than risking them).
- Collective, successful navigation ensures future growth for the sector, and digital global health's ability to make lives better rather than worse.

General findings and recommendations, summarized below:

- Countries should develop holistic national digital health strategies. There is wide disparity in progress in this area among LMICs, with several important countries having no formal national plans. Digital technologies will not achieve anywhere near their full potential absent a plan that provides the necessary resources, coordination, cooperation, and leadership. These plans need to be holistic, in part, as each country's situation will be somewhat different, including the considerable complexity that comes from integrating digital technologies with legacy health systems.
- Several multilateral organizations and private-sector initiatives have elevated the focus on digital health at the international level, such as the WHO-backed global digital health strategy. LMICs should work with WHO and other actors to mobilize the resources and expertise to help develop and implement—or improve—their own digital health strategies.
- Training and education to use digital technologies is critical, but few LMICs have integrated digital skills into their health-workforce training. Regional and multilateral health organizations, donors, and other stakeholders should prioritize efforts to help LMICs address the most pressing skills gaps.
- There are particularly acute gaps in ICT infrastructure in LMICs, which are home to most of the people that remain disconnected from the Internet. Poor ICT infrastructure severely limits the potential of digital health. Regional and multilateral development agencies, and other donors, should fill these gaps to cover private-sector shortfalls—for example, with regard to wireless mobile coverage in rural areas.

- LMICs need to enact a data governance framework that balances data privacy and protection with innovation. The generation, protection, use, sharing, and international transfer of high-quality data is fundamental to an effective and innovative digital health program. An overly restrictive data governance framework will limit the potential of digital health technologies.
- Policymakers need to build interoperability into their frameworks from the start, as many of the benefits of digital health technologies require cross-border transfers of data. This is critical, as many firms and research organizations involved in digital health rely on the Internet, the free flow of data, and centralized IT facilities to easily, cheaply, and reliably access data, patients, and health-care providers around the world. The emergence of a meaningful, integrated global digital health framework will depend on national governments enabling cross-border flows of data.

Digital technologies offer unique opportunities to strengthen health systems, as illustrated once more by the COVID19 pandemic, when the use and oftentimes remarkably fast deployment of various digital tools and solutions has allowed countries to better detect and prevent the spread as well as to respond to the pandemic. In general, digital health technologies can help meet the challenge of both the changing health needs of the public and the ever tighter fiscal space.

In the health sector, the potential benefits of digital technologies are abundant. Ensuring access to the right information by the right people at the right time can improve safety, effectiveness, and efficiency of care. Digitally enhanced health services can improve access and help move away from reactive towards proactive approaches to preserving health. Health workers could be relieved from time consuming routine tasks and interact better with patients. Patients could become more engaged, improve self care skills, and more effectively coproduce health.

However, despite some isolated successes as well as the recent acceleration in uptake of digital technologies achieved during the COVID19 pandemic, the health sector is a long way behind other industries in reaping digital opportunities. Investment in technical infrastructure plays an important role and is often insufficient, but even an ideal technical infrastructure will not guarantee a success.

Successful digital transformation in the health sector is not a simple matter of technical change but requires a complex adaptive change in human attitudes and skills as well as in the organization of work and the related legal and financial frameworks. Digital technologies only provide the tools and cannot transform the health sector on its own but need to be put to productive use by the health workers and patients.

Digital health is frequently only available as an elective course in education or professional training programmes and not taught at a high enough level. Moreover, it is presented as a standalone subject rather than being integrated across subjects, which is not conducive to building a digital culture or the perception of digital technologies as an integral component of health services.

This calls for ensuring the presence of digital health in the core content of education and professional training as well as investment in creating modern and comprehensive digital health curricula for future and current health workers. The curricula should not only focus on skills for merely operating digital tools, but also on skills such as critical appraisal of information and digital health ethics.

To meet the current demand for digital upskilling more systematic support should be created that ensures up-skilling for all categories of health workers, in particular through more flexible (self) learning opportunities. The prevailing problems of Continuous Professional Development (CPD) and other professional training systems, such as a lack of dedicated time or means for up-skilling on the part of health workers, need to be also addressed.

Addressing the critical challenges of digital transformation requires policy makers and technologists as well as clinical leaders/managers and technologists to work together and understand more of each other's fields. However, health systems lack clinician leaders and managers with a combined understanding of clinical practice, technology, and change management. There is also evidence of a deficit of informaticians and system optimisers with strong insights into health care.

This requires more of the joint degree and hybrid educational programmes that combine the understanding of, for example, clinical practice, technology, and change management or health policy, ethics, and technology. The programmes at the executive and postgraduate levels should attract professionals who are already pursuing a career in, for example, clinical practice or digital technology.

Digital transformation is critically dependent not only on the increasingly widespread presence of digital tools and solutions in the health sector, but also on whether their presence results in the development of new forms of cooperation and models for how health services are provided. The new ways of working, however, might not fit within the existing legal, financial, or organizational frameworks, which need to be adapted such that the health systems can quickly start using novel solutions.

New digitally enabled health services, for example, need to be adequately recognised in provider payment systems. Similarly, if digital technology augments health workers' tasks and roles, regulations need to timely allow for expanding or reassigning these tasks and roles. The implementation of digital technologies by health care organizations needs to be planned, as, in most cases, it takes a considerable amount of time of frontline health workers, which must be accounted for and allowed for.

THE FUTURE OF DIGITAL HEALTH

To help cope with the social distancing measures put in place to help flatten the curve of COVID-19 infections, the healthcare industry had to adapt quickly. Digital health became a saving grace for hospitals, clinics and doctors at the height of the pandemic in search of a way to provide the same quality of care services while minimizing the spread of the coronavirus. Key trends have emerged surrounding the use of the technology that will continue to shape the future of digital health services.

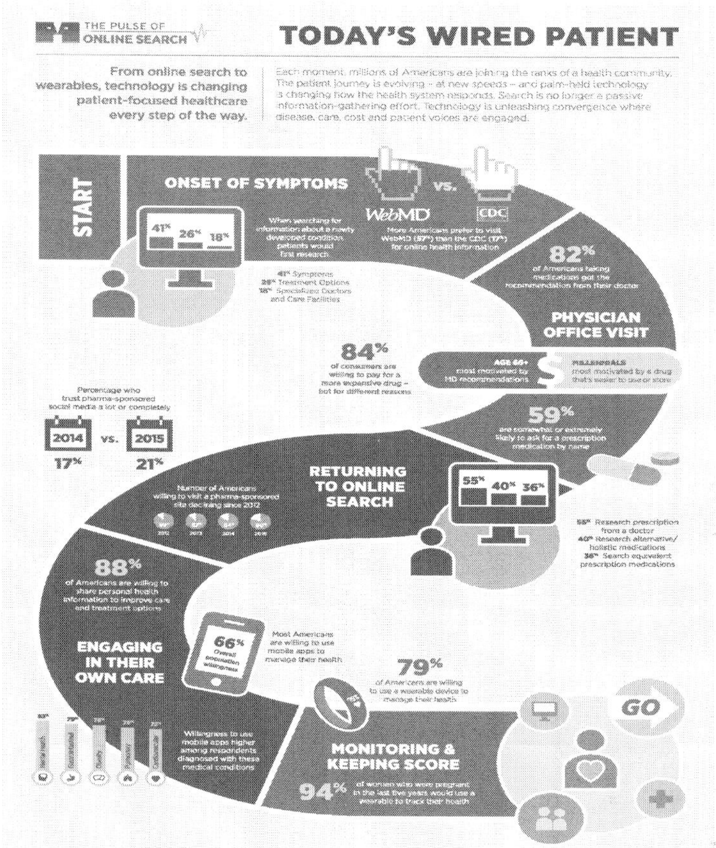

Figure 36. Today's wired patient.

Source: Makovsky 2022

Simply put, digital health uses communication technology to deliver healthcare services to patients without the need to be in the same physical location such as video chat via apps or webcams, phones, or video conference software (NEJM, 2018). Prior to the pandemic, digital health services were generally limited adhoc services with a large range of restrictions (Pennic, 2020). Originally, they were created to support rural and underserved patients gain access to specialists when local help was severely limited (Rutledge et al., 2017). Jump forward to 2020-2021, and digital health is becoming widespread across all aspects of the industry.

According to the Centers for Disease Control and Prevention (CDC), digital health utilization spiked by more than 154% in late March of 2020 compared to the same period in 2019 (Koonin et al., 2020). Additionally, the market is expected to rise to over $397 billion USD by 2027 following current predictions made by Fortune Business Insight (Fortune Business Insights, 2021). To illustrate the impact the pandemic has had on the industry, in 2019 the market was only worth $42 billion USD.5While usage over time has subsided since the peak of the pandemic, it has become clear that digital health is now an instrumental part of the future of healthcare delivery (Bestsenny et al., 2020).

1. Increased patient utilization

What originally was implemented as a strategy to reduce the amount of community transmission, has led to an active conversation between healthcare professionals about the continuation of digital health consultations for many clients in the future. It is now considered a cost-effective first line of treatment for non-urgent and follow-up appointments.

As of July 2021, digital health utilization has stabilized at 38 times higher than pre-pandemic levels.6 And, even pre-pandemic, evidence supported the increased use of digital health (AMA, 2020). In a survey conducted by McKinsey, 76% of patients said they would be interested in using digital health moving forward (Bestsenny et al., 2020). Furthermore, over half of respondents in a study from the Journal of Telemedicine and Telecare said they would utilize digital health to; refill medications, prepare for an upcoming visit, review test results, or receive education (Ebbert et al., 2021). We can expect to see healthcare providers and insurance companies working together moving forward to broaden the availability and accessibility of digital health.

2. Increased chronic care management

Approximately 1 in 3 of all adults suffer from a chronic condition globally, which includes, kidney disease, heart disease, cancer, lung disease, alzhemiers, diabetes and stroke side effects (Hajat et al., 2018). In most cases lifestyle choices and preventative care methods can help these patients prevent and treat these diseases (Willet et al., 2006). However, a large portion of these patients do not follow through with their treatment, do not take or refill their repeat prescriptions, or do not attend their regular follow-up appointments to help manage their symptoms (Brown et al., 2011).

This lack of adherence to a care plan costs the industry billions a year (Luga et al., 2014). Digital health has the potential to not only reduce the cost of a care plan, but also improve patient engagement and adherence to it. Digital health is a convenient way for patients to connect to their doctor quickly and frequently. Removing the need for lengthy waits in waiting rooms, and the cost of continuous commutes to the doctors' office. Additionally, having more frequent connections between patients and doctors may allow for small problems to be caught early enough to reduce the risk of further problems or complications.

3. Greater focus on mental health

Just over 10% of people globally suffer from mental health disorders (Ritchie et al., 2018). The pandemic only seemed to worsen the situation causing an increase in depression and anxiety as a result of lockdowns, isolations and the fear of the unknown increase. According to the World Health Organization (WHO), the COVID-19 pandemic disrupted mental health services in 93% of countries worldwide (WHO, 2020). Those already receiving treatment saw their support groups close, their appointments canceled with the clinics, and their outlets for alleviating symptoms became severely limited.

In order to continue to treat patients many therapists, counselors and doctors quickly turned to video conferencing to continue to support their patients. Hence the development of teletherapy and telepsychiatry began and moving forward, this will likely become a widely accepted form of treatment. Without the pandemic, it is still thought that only about half of those diagnosed with mental health disorders receive treatment (National Institute of Mental Health, 2021). This is partially due to the limited availability of specialists in one given area, but thanks to the progression of teletherapy and telepsychiatry, this will hopefully be a thing of the past.

4. Improved user experience

Patient demand has been the greatest driving force when it comes to the growth in digital health. This demand for convenient access to care services will continue and as a result, a greater expectation will be placed on providers. As organizations plan for the future of digital health, patient experience and expectations should be at the forefront of their minds (Kreofsky, 2020). Additionally, as this demand continues to rise, more and more companies are branching out and entering the market and hence organizations will need to do something to put themselves ahead of the competition.

Patients want their digital health experience to be seamless and integrated, nobody wants to have to juggle multiple different apps and websites. This means developers are looking at ways to ensure comprehensive service through integrated communications such as video, webchat, and bots, while allowing for real-time updates, reminders and follow-up appointments

(Griffin, 2021). On top of this it must be streamlined for easy use, allowing patients to access and navigate all their information at the touch of a button.

5. Integrated data sharing

It is not new that services that allow data sharing are easier and more convenient to use and as a result, this is the direction that digital health is heading. Many digital health apps are beginning to utilize and communicate with fitness apps, for example, to gather information regarding step count, and heart rate directly from an individual's devices. This will give healthcare professionals a more rounded view of a person's lifestyle, and paired with electronic healthcare records, can help create a clearer picture of their current health (Griffin, 2021).

This idea of integrated data sharing is being driven by interoperability, which is the ability to access, exchange, integrate and cooperatively use data in a coordinated manner, within and across different organizations timely and effectively (Chan, 2021). When systems are interoperable they not only share the data but can interpret the data and present it as its received, preserving its original context (Chan, 2021). This is the future of digital health and providers need to move from just providing and recording facts to passing on these critical insights back to maximize the benefits to the patients.

6. Wearable technology and remote patient monitoring

As stated previously, digital health is becoming vital for those with chronic conditions and with that the idea of integrated data sharing leads to the next trend for the future and that is wearable technology. Wearable technology has been around for decades going back to 1970 when HP created a calculator wristwatch. Fast forward to 2009, the first Fitbit fitness tracker was developed (Thilen, 2020). Enter the Apple Watch in 2015, which further enhanced the development and growth in product sales of smartwatches and fitness trackers (Thilen, 2020). This has allowed the healthcare industry to easily and efficiently begin remote patient monitoring (Phaneuf, 2021). These devices allow doctors to gather real-time data on a number of health measures including activity levels, heart rates, blood pressure, sleep cycles, and glucose levels, more directly from their patients.

Armed with all this additional data about a typical day in the life of their patients, doctors will be able to make more insightful diagnoses and recommendations. Integrating these devices with a secure digital health platform and electronic health records, will allow members of care teams to intervene at the first sign of trouble. With that said, there will likely be an increase in wearable technology and the sharing of data generated by these devices with healthcare providers, on the condition that patients trust the security and privacy measures in place. Furthermore, the technology and platforms must be easy to use to ensure easy integration into daily life for the patient and doctor (Pennic, 2020).

7. Convenient remote pediatric care

Monitoring a sick child is never easy. Children are often good at masking their symptoms, have difficulty communicating and often become shy or scared in front of medical staff (Cootes, 2010). This becomes especially difficult for those who need long-term monitoring. But, with the use of digital health, it becomes more convenient for the parent and can lower the costs of high-quality care (Utidjian et al., 2016).

Pre-pandemic pediatric digital health was already seeing growth, but it is thought that this growth will become more widespread in the next few years. This is thanks to the upcoming generations of parents becoming more accustomed to using virtual technology than previous generations (Yarnell., 2020). In addition, there is an increase in digital health services being directed toward young people, for example, the development of virtual physiotherapy designed to mimic video games (Kumari et al., 2020). Overall, it is likely that the adoption of digital health for pediatric care will continue to grow significantly over the next few years (Curfman et al., 2021).

8. Investments in technology

Finally, digital health will not be possible without the technological infrastructure to support it, and as a result, further investments need to be made. The use of digital health tools is ever-evolving, from COVID-19 Tracing apps, to wellness trackers to digital health and virtual health apps – all of which are accessible from the comfort of home (Chan et al., 2020). In terms of digital health, investments in knowledge and technology will enable more effective initiatives and applications.6 digital health encompasses a shift toward a more effective, patient-centric approach both in terms of providing targeted and responsive levels of care where patients prefer, as well as reducing pressures on the healthcare workforce (Chan et al., 2020).

There are not enough healthcare professionals and there has been a labor shortage for some time, which was highlighted during the pandemic (Chan et al., 2021). Investments into technology that supports the growth in digital health, will further reduce pressure on the workforce and potentially allow them to deliver better care.

These are the key trends that have become clear since the widespread adoption of digital health services over the last 18 months. Digital health provides the healthcare industry with so many advantages that although we are starting to see the end of this pandemic, the utilization of this revolutionary technology will continue far into the future.

Digital health has proved not only to be more convenient for patients but it has the potential to provide so many further benefits including improving public health, improving access to care, relieving pressure on the healthcare workforce, and helping to reduce financial stress.

Digital health has been the saving grace for the healthcare industry during the pandemic, but as we begin to move forward, what is clear is that digital health is here to stay.

CHALLENGES FACED BY THE DIGITAL HEALTH INDUSTRY

There are substantial challenges that the digital health industry faces that must be considered within any insurance and liability analysis:

- Regulatory and legal frameworks that cannot keep pace within innovation, adoption and use.
- Consumer concerns about security and privacy.
- Ethical questions that inevitably arise in the adoption and use of new technologies, especially regarding the role of commercialism and monetization.
- Interoperability issues and fragmented systems –both technical (software, platforms etc.) and 'system structure' (e.g. disparate providers, payors and regulators of healthcare).
- Competing motivations and misalignments – payor, provider and patient (what are the priorities and how can they be agreed upon).
- Equity issues that can especially arise from swift digital implementations – e.g. digital literacy issues, digital access issues ('digital divide') and the impact on vulnerable groups (e.g. seniors – the 'grey divide').
- Usability issues for patients and providers alike.

There are a multiplicity of activities, entities and thus corresponding exposures and harms that can arise in digital health contexts:

- Providers using, developing or implementing digital health technologies to facilitate patient interactions (diagnosis, treatment, monitoring and management).
- Digital health platform hosts, developers and designers (software, applications, hardware), especially those that facilitate or provide patient diagnosis treatment, monitoring and management.
- Product manufacturers, distributors, developing digital health technologies (both regulated and unregulated).

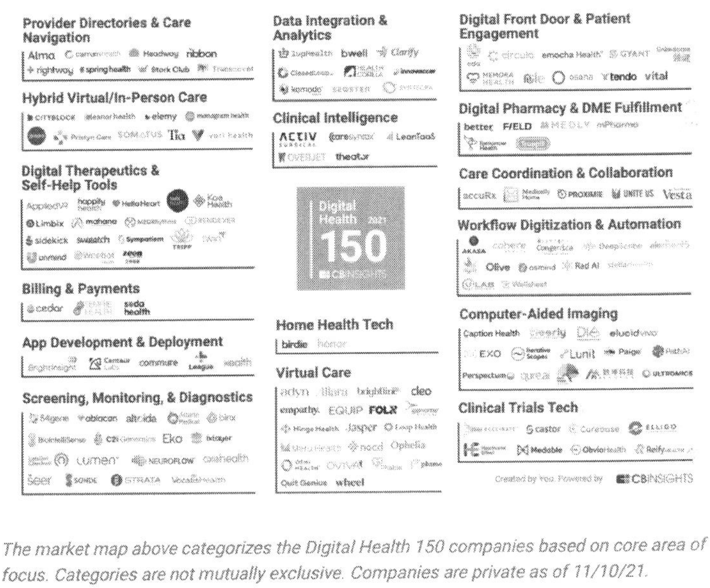

Figure 37. The Top Digital Health Companies Of 2021.

Source: CB Insights 2021

RISING TRENDS IN DIGITAL HEALTH

Healthcare and technology go hand-in-hand. But the question on many people's minds is where are they going? Digital health trends like telemedicine, IoT devices, and virtual reality surgical training continue to attract massive investment, helping the industry improve health equity worldwide.

The World Health Organization defines health equity as "... the absence of unfair and avoidable or remediable differences in health among population groups defined socially, economically, demographically or geographically."

Put simply, health equity is all about making healthcare more accessible and affordable for everyone — and digital health trends are the driving forces behind health equity.

Of course, there are many challenges on the road to achieving this goal, with stakeholders at all levels of government involved and a myriad of social determinants of how we collect, analyze, and share health data.

Read on as we explore the five crucial digital health trends in 2021 and explain why they matter to health equity and the future of healthcare.

5 Biggest Digital Health Trends to Watch

The pandemic triggered massive disruption in the healthcare industry and pushed the sector to invest more in innovative new technology. Some of the following digital health trends gained momentum during the pandemic and are predicted to change the future of medicine:

1. TELEHEALTH

Telehealth is the use of digital communication technologies such as computers, mobile phones, and tablets, to facilitate the delivery of healthcare services.

As social distancing reduced in-person visits, healthcare providers had to pivot quickly. By April 2020, over 43% of Medicare primary care visits were conducted via telehealth services.

Even as the COVID-19 vaccines roll out globally, telehealth looks set to stay. Studies from Fortune Business Insights predict the telehealth market will grow beyond $185 billion by 2026.

Why it matters:

Telehealth offers multiple benefits, including:

- Expanded healthcare access: More people can access health-related services, including medically vulnerable people and people without transportation or a provider in their local area.
- Reduced contact: There is less contact between healthcare workers and patients, and also less chance of illness spreading, with fewer patients in medical buildings.

- Care for urgent non-COVID-19 conditions: Patients with chronic conditions who need frequent checkups may be able to schedule remote appointments, if no in-person tests are required.
- Continuity of care: With consistent communication, providers can nurture their relationships with patients and potentially avoid any negative consequences caused by delayed or missed in-person appointments.

What to expect:

People want a seamless digital experience to schedule appointments, get medication, and receive essential communication and advice on their health. Telehealth — instead of being a passing trend — is expected to become an important component of a comprehensive health care plan that improves the patient experience.

An estimated 40% of primary care appointments could be conducted remotely, and providers that offer telehealth options are likely to benefit from greater patient volume. The American Hospital Association reported that hospitals lost $161.4 billion from March to June 2020. Telehealth could help hospitals recoup some of those losses.

McKinsey estimates that $250 billion of the total U.S. healthcare spend may go virtual in the years after the pandemic. Rather than looking to digital health trends as an experimental option, the sector must fully embrace innovation to improve the agility and efficiency of providers in the future.

2. IOT AND MEDICINE

The Internet of Things (IoT) is the growing network of physical objects that contain software, sensors, and other technologies that enable connections and data exchanges with disparate devices and systems across the internet.

Medical IoT is a rapidly growing field that uses wearable devices, monitors, and integrated applications for healthcare needs. With AI and machine learning technology, medical IoT can offer enhanced versions of traditional medical devices, like the smart inhaler — a device that syncs patient usage with a mobile app.

Why it matters:

Medical IoT offers multiple benefits, including:

- Remote monitoring: Patients can use wearable devices and go about their lives. Meanwhile, healthcare professionals can remotely monitor patients' conditions with real-time data insights, reducing the frequency of in-person appointments

- Improved convenience: With the rise of 5G and smart technology in healthcare, patients have more ability to manage their conditions and health needs. For example, smart insulin pens, and glucose monitoring devices help people keep tabs on their health needs with minimal disruption to their lives.
- Lower costs for patients: As the technology improves, many IoT devices will become more affordable, edging us closer to health equity. That's good news for patients.
- Lower costs for hospitals: Hospitals rely on their complex medical equipment, such as X-ray machines, CAT scanners, and magnetic resonance imagers (MRI). The cost of replacing one of those machines is exorbitant, and any amount of machine downtime is costly. With IoT devices that monitor these machines and alert technicians about problems, hospitals can perform better predictive maintenance and avoid costly downtime.
- Furthermore, hospitals can use sensors to track supply inventory, optimizing their usage and spending on gases, chemicals, and disposable items like masks, gloves, and syringes.

What to expect:

IoT is one of the fastest-growing digital health trends of 2021 — DataProt reports a compound annual growth rate (CAGR) of 28.6% this year. This growth is supported by the global adoption of cloud computing and mobile apps.

When it comes to healthcare, data storage and security are paramount. Patients must be able to trust healthcare providers with sensitive personal information. In addition to protecting personal information, IoT devices must be reliable in terms of their connections, performance, and real-time data delivery. If there are any lags or downtime, healthcare professionals could miss critical information about a patient's health.

The cloud age is ripe with opportunities for healthcare, but trust in data security and IoT functionality is still evolving. With that in mind, we can expect greater investment and funding to improve upon IoT technology in the years ahead.

3. APPS FOR EMPLOYEE WELLNESS

As the harsh reality of lockdown life sank in, 2020 brought untold mental health challenges for people across the world. Suddenly, mindfulness apps like Headspace, Liberate, and Calm weren't just for the niche meditation audience, as mainstream adoption drove download numbers in the wellness app market. According to a report from The New York Times, Calm acquired 10 million new users, and venture capitalists pooled

$75 million to take the company's valuation north of $2 billion.

Employers are increasingly recognizing that wellness apps could be helpful for their employees. Company initiatives like corporate wellness retreats, workplace yoga, and team-building events have been around for decades, but the employer-provided wellness app is a relatively new concept.

Why it matters:

Employee wellness apps offer multiple benefits, including:

- Increased job satisfaction: A report from SHRM found that 48% of U.S. employees claim that they would have more confidence in digital health tools if their employer offered them. Moreover, 26% said that if such apps were on offer, they would be more inclined to stay with their current employer.
- Reduced costs: The increasing usage of health apps will help reduce overall health costs for providers and patients. In 2018, reports estimated health apps might save the U.S. healthcare system $7 billion each year. As the mobile age continues to attract more people to wellness apps, employers should see a decrease in employee "sick days," which would in turn boost productivity.
- Personalized healthcare: Many health and wellness apps enable users to set up a personal profile, which will then track key measures like weight, calorie count, and blood sugar levels. With personalized healthcare at our fingertips, people can have more control over their health. Also, users can share health data with their providers.

What to expect:

Some of the apps targeting the corporate workplace include Limeade, which enables companies to nurture a culture of well-being and inclusion, and Vantage Fit, which helps employers create simple wellness programs and challenges to help their employees stay fit and healthy.

The Future of Health report from Deloitte projects wellness to continue as one of the most important digital health trends in the next 20 years. By 2040, we can expect a fundamental shift away from treatment-focused medicine, with 60% of spending going toward improving health and well-being.

In line with this trend, employers will focus more on marketing to audiences that are interested in wellness apps and practices. Companies will implement digital wellness strategies as they attempt to build their teams and improve workplace morale and job satisfaction.

4. CONTINUED INNOVATIONS IN INFECTIOUS DISEASE MANAGEMENT

Soon after the COVID-19 pandemic began, it was apparent just how unprepared the healthcare sector was to handle the situation. Within a few weeks, the only digital health trends worth talking about were those that sought to combat the spread of the virus.

Many countries raced to launch apps that would help governments and healthcare providers with virus testing, tracking, and monitoring. No sooner than one app was launched, another would arrive with enhanced capabilities for shorter testing times and better tracking features.

Unfortunately, it took the tragedy of the pandemic to spark innovation in the healthcare industry. While there have been massive losses since the end of 2019, there has also been tremendous progress.

Why it matters:

There have been remarkable breakthroughs in genomics and sequencing technologies In the last two decades. This progress laid the foundation for the COVID-19 vaccines and made their accelerated development possible.

Messenger RNA (mRNA) is the basis of the first vaccines. But it's not limited to tackling COVID-19, as it enables researchers to create many other vaccines and treatments at much lower costs and in less time than traditional methods. Described as "biological software," mRNA vaccines can be customized with a protein code that stimulates an immune response to a specific pathogen.

We may soon see new solutions for other diseases, including malaria, hepatitis B, tuberculosis, and cystic fibrosis. Furthermore, researchers are looking at how mRNA medicines could be used to treat cancer, with clinical trials in progress.

What to expect:

The rapid innovation in healthcare throughout 2020 made it possible to bring testing for COVID-19 mobile. Soon, we should be able to test for other infectious diseases outside of traditional healthcare settings, enabling providers to test people in workplaces, schools, and homes.

In February 2021, Moderna, Inc. announced intentions to ramp up manufacturing investment, as it targets the production of 1.4 billion doses of its COVID-19 vaccine in 2022. We can also assume that virtual healthcare will enhance efforts to control the spread of disease.

Historically, the vaccine development process has been slow — 10 years, in some cases — but production timelines for mRNA vaccines could be as short as three to four months.

In the future, AI and predictive analytics will be crucial to helping medical professionals develop a better scientific understanding of the incubation and spread of infectious diseases. However, at a more fundamental level, the entire global health system is set for an overhaul of supply chains and logistics so that it's possible to deliver effective, affordable vaccines and healthcare to whoever needs it when they need it. '

5. VIRTUAL AND AUGMENTED REALITY

Not long ago, virtual reality seemed like a novelty best suited to video games. Now, virtual reality (VR) and augmented reality (AR) technology offer a wide range of practical uses beyond gaming and entertainment.

In healthcare, VR helps with surgical training and planning, enabling both surgeons and patients to get more comfortable with procedures. There are also many reports about the efficacy of VR for helping with chronic pain management and mental health.

MarketsandMarkets conducted a study on the expected growth of AR and VR in healthcare, projecting a 30.7% annual growth rate between 2017 and 2025.

Why it matters:

Health professionals already use virtual reality to treat a variety of conditions, including mental illnesses, such as anxiety, phobias, and post-traumatic stress disorder. Providers can use VR and AR technology to create simulations of real-life scenarios where people feel psychologically challenged — for example, dealing with eating disorders, a fear of heights, or social anxiety.

Although people understand when they put on a VR headset or use an augmented reality application that the environment is artificial, the simulation gives them an opportunity to face challenges and overcome their fear with practice. Oxford VR reports that this style of immersive therapy can reduce fears and phobias by 68% after an average treatment time of only two hours.

On the providers' side, VR helps medical professionals build their skillset. A study on the impact of VR training in healthcare revealed that students who received VR training were able to complete medical procedures 20% faster than a group who only received traditional training. Also, the VR-trained group completed 38% more steps correctly.

What to expect:

The healthcare VR market was just $2 billion in 2019, but a recent report from Verified Market Research predicts massive growth, to the tune of $34 billion by 2027.

In the next year (and beyond), we'll witness many new VR and AR applications in healthcare. These technologies transcend the short shelf life of many digital health trends, as they present tangible long-term benefits for medical professionals and patients, which can save time and money, and improve overall patient care.

Companies like Oxford VR and Karuna Labs are leading a mission to help people who have chronic pain and mental illness — both of which were health problems long before the pandemic lockdown.

VR is still a developing technology. As it continues to advance, its capabilities herald exciting developments for areas like preventive healthcare, rehabilitation, and cancer therapy.

CONCLUSIONS

Information and communication technology can be used to improve the quality and safety of healthcare and to lower costs. But in both developed and developing countries, there is an inadequate supply of skilled individuals who have the technical skills to use this technology to improve health care. Some studies project workforce needs of tens of thousands in English-speaking developed countries, but it is not known what size of workforce will be required in the developing world. It is important to identify and develop the skills, training, and competencies—consistent with local cultures, languages, and health systems—that will be needed to realize the full benefits of these technologies.

When designing an educational or training program, it may not be possible to cover numerous competencies presented in a framework; rather, the program should focus on a specific set of competencies suitable for a particular group of health care workers, role, level of seniority, geographical, and health care setting. However, the identified competency domains prevalent in more than half of the included frameworks (ie, informatics concepts and processes, health information management, communication, ethics, legal, or regulations, and privacy and security) should be considered essential interprofessional competencies and thus should be incorporated into training and education efforts for any health care worker group. In addition, several digital competencies presented in the included frameworks may already be covered within the existing curriculum. For example, competencies within the *Analysis* and *Research* category may have been integrated within epidemiology training and evidence-based medicine education, respectively. Therefore, educators should consider integrating digital health training within existing parts of the curriculum and teaching it in an applied manner as much as possible.

As countries seek to strengthen their healthcare systems while adapting to continuously evolving demands, there is a unique opportunity to embed such digital, data-driven practices into everyday healthcare operations, and to rethink how and where care is delivered. Patients are asking for it. Growing staff shortages demand it. And technology enables it.

The transition into the Digital Age provides novel opportunities to minimize existing inequalities and pursue the Agenda for Sustainable Development. However, to effectively pursue this goal, we must first ensure that inequalities are not exacerbated during this transition. Based on the current findings, we conclude that Europe's digital climate at the start of the pandemic left much to be desired, showcasing large in- and cross-country discrepancies in internet access and digital skills. Although the pandemic forced society to digitalise, it remains to be seen how much sticks around. One conclusion, however, is certain: Europe cannot be considered a homogenous zone in terms of internet access or digital skills and pursuing a complete digital transition would currently exacerbate in- and cross-country inequalities.

REFERENCES

1. Abbas J, Wang D, Su Z, Ziapour A (2021). The Role of Social Media in the Advent of COVID-19 Pandemic: Crisis Management, Mental Health Challenges and Implications. Risk Manag Healthc Policy. 12;14:1917–32. pmid:34012304
2. Academy of Medical Royal Colleges (2011). E Health Competency Framework - Defining the Role of the Expert Clinician. Available from: https://www.physio-pedia.com/images/f/f0/EHealth_Competancy_Framework.pdf. Accessed 18.03.2022
3. Adam M, McMahon SA, Prober C, Bärnighausen T (2019). Human-centered design of video-based health education: an iterative, collaborative, community-based approach. J Med Internet Res 30;21(1):e12128
4. Adellund HK. (2016). eSundhedskompetence og brugsmønstre af eksisterende e-sundhedstilbud hos ambulante medicinske patienter med kroniske sygdomme-spørgeskemaundersøgelse. Available from:: http://2016.e-sundhedsobservatoriet.dk/forslag/patientrapporterede-oplysninger-pro/esundhedskompetence-og-brugsm-nstre-af-eksisterende-e. Accessed 06.04.2022
5. Adler-Milstein J, Kvedar J, Bates DW (2014). digital health among US hospitals: several factors, including state reimbursement and licensure policies, influence adoption. Health Aff (Millwood) 33(2):207-215
6. Adobe XD (2021). Available from: https://www.adobe.com/products/xd.html. Accessed 14.04.2022

7. African Development Working Group (2014). Center for Global Development & The African Population and Health Research Center. Delivering on the Data Revolution in Sub-Saharan Africa. Washington, D.C.: Center for Global Development & The African Population and Health Research Center. Available from: https://www.cgdev.org/sites/default/files/CGD14-01%20complete%20for%20web%200710.p. Accessed 03.03.2022

8. Agarwal, P., et al. (2019). Mobile App for Improved Self-Management of Type 2 Diabetes: Multicenter Pragmatic Randomized Controlled Trial. JMIR Mhealth Uhealth. 7(1): p. e10321. Available from: https://doi.org/10.2196/10321. Accessed 05.04.2022

9. Ahonen, O., Kouri, P., Liljamo, P., Granqvist, H., Junttila, K., Kinnunen, U. M., Kuurne, S., Numminen, J., Salanterä, S., & Saranto, K. (2015). eHealth Strategy of the Finnish Nurses Association 2015-2020. Finnish Nurses Association eHealth Expert Working Group.

10. Aitken M, Lyle J (2015). Patient Adoption of mHealth, Use, Evidence and Remaining Barriers to Mainstream Acceptance. IMS Institute for Healthcare Informatics. Available from: https://www.iqvia.com/-/media/iqvia/pdfs/institute-reports/patient-adoption-of-mhealth.pdf. Accessed 28.02.2022

11. Ajiboye BA, Adekoya AJ, Alawiye MK, Oyedipe WJ (2014). Knowledge and utilization of health information and communication technologies (HICTs) by health workers of the North-Eastern health zone of Ogun State, Nigeria. *Inform Health Soc Care.* 39:104–23

12. Akanbi MO, Ocheke AN, Agaba PA, Daniyam CA, Agaba EI, Okeke EN, et al (2012). Use of electronic health records in sub-Saharan Africa: Progress and challenges. *J Med Trop.* 14:1–6

13. Alam K, Oliveras E (2014). Retention of female volunteer community health workers in Dhaka urban slums: a prospective cohort study. Hum Resour Health. 12:29.

14. Allam Z, Jones DS (2020). On the Coronavirus (COVID-19) outbreak and the Smart City Network: Universal data sharing standards coupled with artificial intelligence (AI) to benefit urban health monitoring and management. Healthcare (Basel). 8(1)

15. Allen B, Seltzer SE, Langlotz CP, Dreyer KP, Summers RM, Petrick N, et al. (2019). A road map for translational research on artificial intelligence in medical imaging: From the 2018 National

Institutes of Health/RSNA/ACR/The Academy Workshop. J Am Coll Radiol 16(9 Pt A):1179-89

16. Almeida F, Duarte Santos J, Augusto Monteiro J (2020). The Challenges and Opportunities in the Digitalization of Companies in a Post-COVID-19 World. IEEE Eng Manag Rev. 48(3):97–103
17. American Medical Association. (2020). Available from https://www.ama-assn.org/system/files/2020-02/ama-digital-health-study.pdf. Accessed 20.04.2022
18. Archer N. (2011). Project Management Characteristics and Education for eHealth Students. EJHI 6(4):e30
19. Aungst TD, Patel R (2020). Integrating digital health into the curriculum-considerations on the current landscape and future developments. J Med Educ Curric Dev 2020;7:2382120519901275
20. Australian Health Informatics Education Council (2011). Health Informaticscope, Careers and Competencies. Available from: https://www.ahiec.org.au/docs/AHIEC_HI_Scope_Careers_and_Competencies_V1-9.pdf. Accessed 16.03.202
21. Awokola BI, Abioye-Kuteyi EA, Ogundele OA, Awokola EO (2011). Computer and internet use by doctors in a Nigerian Teaching Hospital: A survey of the wesley guild unit of Obafemi Awolowo University Teaching Hospitals complex. *Middle East J Fam Med.* 9:17–21.
22. Awokola BI, Abioye-Kuteyi EA, Otoru OO, Oyegbade OO, Awokola EO, Awokola OA, et al (2012). Practical challenges of setting up an electronic medical record system in a Nigerian tertiary hospital: The wesley guild hospital experience. *Middle East J Fam Med.* 7:37–42
23. Ayres EJ, Greer-Carney JL, Fatzinger McShane PE, Miller A, Turner P (2012). Nutrition informatics competencies across all levels of practice: a national Delphi study. J Acad Nutr Diet 112(12):2042-2053
24. Baldwin, J. L., Singh, H., Sittig, D. F., & Giardina, T. D. (2016). Patient portals and health apps: Pitfalls, promises, and what one might learn from the other symptoms. Healthcare, 5 (3), 81–85
25. Bandura A (1977). Self-efficacy: Towards a unifying theory of behavioral change. Psychological Review 84; 2, 191-215, 10.1037/0033-295X.84.2.191
26. Bandura A (1992). Self-efficacy: Thought control of action; Schwarzer, Ralf, Eds.; Routledge: Oxon, U.K. pp. 3-38

27. Barakat A, Woolrych RD, Sixsmith A, Kearns WD, Kort HS (2013). eHealth Technology Competencies for Health Professionals Working in Home Care to Support Older Adults to Age in Place: Outcomes of a Two-Day Collaborative Workshop. Med 05;2(2):e10

28. Bautista JR (2015). From solving a health problem to achieving quality of life: redefining eHealth literacy. J Lit Technol 16(2):33-54

29. Benwell N, Hird K, Thomas N, Furness E, Fear M, Sweetman G. (2017). Effectiveness and efficiency of training in digital healthcare packages: training doctors to use digital medical record keeping software. Aust Health Rev 41(5):479-84

30. Bestsenny et al. (2020). Article available from https://www.mckinsey.com/industries/healthcare-systems-and-services/our-insights/telehealth-a-quarter-trillion-dollar-post-covid-19-reality. Accessed 20.04.2022

31. Bhavnani SP, Narula J, Sengupta PP. (2016). Mobile technology and the digitization of healthcare. Eur Heart J. 37(18):1428-38

32. Biggins D, Holley D, Zezulkova M. (2017). Digital Competence and Capability Frameworks in Higher Education: Importance of Life-long Learning, Self-Development and Well-being. EAI Endorsed Transactions on e-Learning 4(13):e1

33. Blak R, Shaw T, Blake A, Hübner U, Kaye R, Schug S, et al. (2016). Healthcare Information and Management Systems Society Foundation. EU-US eHealth Works to Improve Global Workforce Development. Available from: http://www.himss.org/sites/ himssorg/files/eu-us-ehealth-workforce-development.pdf. Accessed 12.02.2022

34. Blake A, Kaye R. (2015). A Digital Solution to the EU/US Skilled eHealth/Health IT Worker Shortage: The HITCOMP Tool and Repository. : EU-US Workforce Development Workgroup. Presented at: eHealth Week; May 11-13, 2015; Riga, Latvia. Available from: https://www.eiseverywhere.com/file_uploads/. Accessed 12.02.2022

35. Blaya JA, Fraser HS, Holt B (2010). E-health technologies show promise in developing countries. *Health Aff (Millwood)* 29:244–51

36. Blondel VD (2013). Data for Development: The D4D Challenge on Mobile Phone Data. *arXiv*. Available from: https://arxiv.org/pdf/1210.0137.pdf. Accessed 03.03.2022

37. Borell, J. (2016). eHealth and work environment –a question of humans, not computers. In G. Erlingsdóttir, & H. Sandberg (Eds.), eHealth opportunities and challenges: A white paper (pp. 36–41).

38. Botts N and Horan T (2008). Bridging care communication health management within diverse underserved populations. 2008 Jan 01 Presented at: Americas Conference on Information Systems. Toronto, ON, Canada

39. Brice S, Almond H (2020). Health Professional Digital Capabilities Frameworks: A Scoping Review. Journal of Multidisciplinary Healthcare 2020, ume 13, 1375-1390, 10.2147/jmdh.s269412.

40. Britt RK, Hatten KN. (2016). The Development and Validation of the eHealth Competency Scale: A Measurement of Self-Efficacy, Knowledge, Usage, and Motivation. Tech Commun Q 07;25(2):137-150

41. Brown et al. (2011). Mayo Clinical Proceedings 86, 304-314

42. Brown, J., Pope, N., Bosco, A. M., Mason, J., & Morgan, A. (2020). Issues affecting nurses' capability to use digital technology at work: An integrative review. Journal of Clinical Nursing, 29 (15–16), 2801–2819

43. Brunie A, Wamala-Mucheri P, Otterness C, Akol A, Chen M, Bufumbo L,

44. Burki T (2019). A milestone on the journey to a digital NHS. Lancet Digital Health. 1(3):e114-5

45. Car J, Lang B, Colledge A, Ung C, Majeed A. (2011). Interventions for enhancing consumers' online health literacy. Cochrane Database Syst Rev (6):CD007092

46. Castelnuovo B, Kiragga A, Afayo V, Ncube M, Orama R, Magero S, et al (2012). Implementation of provider-based electronic medical records and improvement of the quality of data in a large HIV program in Sub-Saharan Africa. *PLoS One.* 7:e51631

47. Castro D and Korte T (2014). Comments to the Senate Finance Committee on Health Data Transparency. The Center for Data Innovation. Available from: http://www2.datainnovation.org/2014-senate-finance-health-data.pdf. Accessed 28.02.2022

48. Catwell L, Sheikh A (2009). Evaluating eHealth interventions: the need for continuous systemic evaluation. PLoS Med Aug;6(8):e1000126

49. Causey M (2014). Medical Device Makers Urged to Play Nicer by Sharing Data. *Quality Digest.* Available from: https://www.

qualitydigest.com/inside/fda-compliance-column/medical-device-makers-urged-play-nicer-sharing-data-021914.html. Accessed 03.03.2022

50. Cellatti F, Wright A, Palen J, Frehywot S, Markus A, Greenberg A, et al. (2010). Can the deployment of community health workers for the delivery of HIV services represent an effective and sustainable response to health workforce shortages? Results of a multicountry study. AIDS. 24:S45–57
51. Chan (2021) Available from https://www.unleashedsoftware.com/blog/8-telehealth-trends-for-2021. Accessed 20.04.2022
52. Chan CV and Kaufman DR (2011). A framework for characterizing eHealth literacy demands and barriers. J Med Internet Res 13(4):e94
53. Chan CV, Matthews LA, Kaufman DR (2009). A taxonomy characterizing complexity of consumer eHealth Literacy. AMIA Annu Symp Proc 14;2009:86-90
54. Chander A, Le UP (2015). Data Nationalism. *Emory Law Journal. Available from:* https://ssrn.com/abstract=2577947. Accessed 05.03.2022
55. Chandrashekar PA (2019). Digital Health Preclinical Requirement for Medical Students. Acad Med. 94(6):749. Available from: http://journals.lww.com/00001888-201906000-00009. Accessed 22.02.2022
56. Chang BL, Bakken S, Brown SS, Houston TK, Kreps GL, Kukafka R, et al (2004). Bridging the digital divide: reaching vulnerable populations. J Am Med Inform Assoc 2004;11(6):448-457
57. Chang J, Poynton MR, Gassert CA, Staggers N (2011). Nursing informatics competencies required of nurses in Taiwan. Int J Med Inform 80(5):332-340
58. Chaplin B, Meloni S, Eisen G, Jolayemi T, Banigbe B, Adeola J, et al (2015). Scale-up of networked HIV treatment in Nigeria: Creation of an integrated electronic medical records system. *Int J Med Inform.* 84:58–68
59. Cheetham, G., & Chivers, G. (1998). The reflective (and competent) practitioner: A model or professional competence which seeks to harmonize the reflective practitioner and competence based approaches. Journal of European Industrial Training, 22 (7), 267– 276

60. Chen CE, Harrington RA, Desai SA, Mahaffey KW, Turakhia MP. (2019). Characteristics of digital health studies registered in ClinicalTrials.gov. JAMA Intern Med. 179(6):838-40
61. Chesser A, Burke A, Reyes J, Rohrberg T (2016). Navigating the digital divide: a systematic review of eHealth literacy in underserved populations in the United States. Inform Health Soc Care 41(1):1-19
62. Chung S and Nahm E (2015). Testing reliability and validity of the eHealth Literacy Scale (eHEALS) for older adults recruited online. Comput Inform Nurs 33(4):150-156
63. Clark N, Becker MH, Janz NK, Lorig K, Rakowski W, Anderson L (1991). Self-Management of Chronic Disease by Older Adults. Journal of Aging and Health. 3 3-27, 10.1177/089826439100300101
64. Cline GB, Luiz JM (2013). Information technology systems in public sector health facilities in developing countries: The case of South Africa. *BMC Med Inform Decis Mak.* 13:13
65. Coiera E (2011). Do we need a national electronic summary care record? Med J Aust. 194(2):90-2
66. Collins FS and Varmus H (2015). A new initiative on precision medicine. N Engl J Med 372(9):793-5
67. Collins S, Yen P, Phillips A, Kennedy MK (2017). Nursing informatics competency assessment for the nurse leader: the delphi study. J Nurs Adm 47(4):212-218
68. Connolly R (2008). Ethical leadership: Training, education, and eLearning to promote ethics as a core competency within the eHealth Program. Ottawa, Canada: Royal Roads University
69. Cootes. (2010). London Journal of Primary Care 3, 19-26
70. Cornwall A and Jewkes R (1995). What is participatory research? Soc Sci Med 41(12):1667-1676
71. Cory N (2017). Cross-Border Data Flows: Where Are the Barriers, and What Do They Cost? Available from: https://itif.org/publications/2017/05/01/cross-border-data-flows-where-are-barriers-and-what-do-they-cost. Accessed 05.03.2022
72. Cory N (2020). Viruses Cross Borders. To Fight Them, Countries Must Let Medical Data Flow, Too. *Innovation Files blogpost.* Available from: https://itif.org/publications/2020/05/07/viruses-cross-borders-fight-them-countries-must-let-medical-data-flow-too. Accessed 05.03.2022

73. Cowan, D. T., Norman, I., & Coopamah, V. P. (2005). Competence in nursing practice: A controversial concept – a focused review of literature. Nurse Education Today, 25, 355– 36
74. Cowhey PF, Aronson JD (2017). Digital DNA: Disruption and the Challenges for Global Governance. New York, NY: Oxford University Press; Available from: https://doi.org/10.1038/nbt.3926 pmid:28787415. Accessed 28.04.2022
75. Crawford A, Sunderji N, López J, Soklaridis S (2016). Defining competencies for the practice of telepsychiatry through an assessment of resident learning needs. BMC Med Educ 26;16:28
76. Curfman A, McSwain SD, Chuo J, et al. Pediatric Telehealth in the COVID-19 Pandemic Era and Beyond. Pediatrics. 2021;148(3):e2020047795
77. Curran CR (2003). Informatics competencies for nurse practitioners. AACN Clin Issues 14(3):320-330
78. Data Driven Development (2015). Pathways for Progress. (Geneva: World Economic Forum. Available from: http://www3.weforum.org/docs/WEFUSA_DataDrivenDevelopment_Report2015.pdf. Accessed 03.03.2022
79. Datiko DG, Lindtjorn B (2010). Cost and cost-effectiveness of smear-positive tuberculosis treatment by health extension workers in Southern Ethiopia: a community randomized trial. PLoS One. 5:e9158
80. de Albuquerque Veloso Machado M, Roberts B, Wong BLH, van Kessel R, Mossialos E (2021). The Relationship Between the COVID-19 Pandemic and Vaccine Hesitancy: A Scoping Review of Literature Until August 2021. Front Public Health. 9:1370. pmid:34650953
81. Deist TM, Dankers FJWM, Ojha P, Scott Marshall M, Janssen T, Faivre-Finn C, et al. (2020). Distributed learning on 20 000+ lung cancer patients - The Personal Health Train. Radiother Oncol. 144:189-200
82. Digi platform (2021). Non-Discriminating Access for Digital Inclusion. Available from: https://izazi.yeboo.com/health_info_dashboard.php. Accessed 14.04.2022
83. DIVI (2020), *DIVI Intensivregister*. Available from: http://dx.doi.org/intensivregister.de. Accessed 04.04.2022
84. Doyle CS. US Department of Education (1992). Outcome Measures for Information Literacy within the National Education Goals of 1990.

Final Report to National Forum on Information Literacy Available from: https://files.eric.ed.gov/fulltext/ED351033. Pdf. Accessed 10.02.2022

85. Duggan F. The Guardian. (2013). Why universities should acquire - and teach - digital literacy Available from: https://www. theguardian. com/education/2013/apr/23/universities-should-teach-digital-literacy. Accessed 10.02.2022
86. Ebbert et al. (2021). Journal of Telemedicine and Telecare. Epub ahead of print
87. Egbert N, Thye J, Hackl WO, Müller-Staub M, Ammenwerth E, Hübner U (2019). Competencies for nursing in a digital world. Methodology, results, and use of the DACH-recommendations for nursing informatics core competency areas in Austria, Germany, and Switzerland. Inform Health Soc Care 44(4):351-375.
88. Egbert N, Thye J, Schulte G, Liebe J, Hackl W, Ammenwerth E, et al (2016). An iterative methodology for developing national recommendations for nursing informatics curricula. Stud Health Technol Inform 228:660-664
89. et al. (2009) Community health workers for ART in sub-Saharan Africa: learning from experience - capitalizing on new opportunities. Hum Resour Health 7:31
90. et al. (2014). Keeping community health workers in Uganda motivated: key challenges, facilitators, and preferred program inputs. Global Health Sci Practice 2:103–16.
91. European Commission (2016). Communication from the Commission to the European Parliament, the Council, the European Economic and Social Committee and the Committee of the Regions: A New Skills Agenda for Europe - Working together to strengthen human capital, employability, and compe [Internet]. 2016. Available from: https://eur-lex.europa.eu/legal-content/EN/TXT/?uri=CELEX:52016DC0381. Accessed 28.04.2022
92. European Commission (2016). The European digital competence framework
93. European Commission (2021). Shaping Europe's digital future: Digital health technologies addressing the pandemic [Internet]. 2021. Available from: https://ec.europa.eu/digital-single-market/en/digital-health-technologies-addressing-pandemic. Accessed 28.04.2022

94. European Commission. European Skills Agenda 2020 (2020). Available from: https://ec.europa.eu/social/main.jsp?catId=1223&langId=en. Accessed 28.04.2022

95. European Medical Students' Association Europe (2019). Digital Health in the Medical Curriculum: Addressing the Needs of the Future Health Workforce. Available from: https://emsa-europe.eu/wp-content/uploads/2019/09/Digital-Health-in-the-Medical-Curriculum_-Addressing-the-Needs-of-the-Future-Health-Workforce.pdf. Accessed 14.03.2022

96. Ezell S, Schultz M, Lund D. (2018). How Innovators Are Solving Global Health Challenges. Available from: https://itif.org/publications/2018/04/24/innovate4health-how-innovators-are-solving-global-health-challenges. Accessed 28.02.2022

97. Farach N, Faba G, Julian S, Mejía F, Cabieses B, D'Agostino M, et al (2015). Stories From the Field: The Use of Information and Communication Technologies to Address the Health Needs of Underserved Populations in Latin America and the Caribbean. JMIR Public Health Surveill. 1(1):e1

98. Federal Ministry of Education and Research (2020), "Wir fördern Nationales Netzwerk der Universitätsmedizin im Kampf gegen Covid19", *Pressemitteilung: 035/2020*. Available from: https://www.bmbf.de/de/karliczekwirfoerdernnationalesnetzwerkder-universitaetsmedizin imkampfgegencovid11230.html. Accessed 04.04.2022

99. Fernandez E, Woldgabreal Y, Day A, Pham T, Gleich B, Aboujaoude E (2021). Live psychotherapy by video versus in-person: A meta-analysis of efficacy and its relationship to types and targets of treatment. Clin Psychol Psychother [Internet]. Available from: https://onlinelibrary.wiley.com/doi/abs/10.1002/cpp.2594 pmid:33826190. Accessed 28.04.2022

100. Fionda B, D'aviero A, Alitto AR, Frascino V, Piras A, Catucci F, et al. (2019). Patient reported outcomes in prostate cancer, a Mobile-Health Essay (PROPHECY). Anticancer Res. (39):1582-3

101. Food and Drug Administration (2018). Framework for FDA's Real-World Evidence Program, Washington, D.C.: U.S. Available from: https://www.fda.gov/media/120060/download. Accessed 03.03.2022

102. for citizens. Publications Office of the European Union

103. Fortune Business Insights. (2021). Available from https://www.fortunebusinessinsights.com/industry-reports/telemedicine-market-101067. Accessed 20.04.2022

104. Fraser HS, Biondich P, Moodley D, Choi S, Mamlin BW, Szolovits P (2005). Implementing electronic medical record systems in developing countries. *Inform Prim Care.* 13:83–95

105. Fridsma DB (2018). Health informatics: a required skill for 21st century clinicians. BMJ. 362:k3043

106. Friedman CP, Donaldson KM, Vantsevich AV (2016). Educating medical students in the era of ubiquitous information. Med Teach 38(5):504-509

107. Gammon D, Berntsen GKR, Koricho AT, Sygna K, Ruland K, Kayser L, Bauer A (2015). The Chronic Care Model and Technological Research and Innovation: A Scoping Review at the Crossroads. Journal of Medical Internet Research 17, e25, 10.2196/jmir.3547

108. Garde D (2014). Big Pharma superteam joins NIH to share data, discover new drugs. *FierceBiotech.* Available from: https://www.fiercebiotech.com/partnering/big-pharma-superteam-joins-nih-to-share-data-discover-new-drugs. Accessed 03.03.2022

109. Gatta R, Vallati M, Dinapoli N, Masciocchi C, Lenkowicz J, Cusumano D, et al. (2019). Towards a modular decision support system for radiomics: A case study on rectal cancer. Artif Intell Med. 96:145-53

110. Gatta R, Vallati M, Lenkowicz J, Casà C, Cellini F, Damiani A, et al. (2018). A framework for event log generation and knowledge representation for process mining in healthcare. In: 30th IEEE International Conference on Tools with Artificial Intelligence (ICTAI 2018) [Internet]. IEEE; 2018 [cited 2019 Apr 18]. p. 647-54. Available from: https://pure.hud.ac.uk/en/publications/a-frame-work-for-event-log-generation-and-knowledge-represen-tation

111. Gilstad H (2014). Toward a comprehensive model of eHealth literacy. Presented at: Practical Aspects of Health Informatics 2014; May 19, 2014; Trondheim, Norway. Available from: http://ceur-ws.org/. Accessed 12.02.2022

112. Gilster P. Digital Literacy. New York, US: John Wiley & Sons, Inc; 1997

113. Global Digital Health Index (2020). Health Enabled and Global Development Incubator. Available from: https://www.digitalhealthindex.org/. Accessed 01.03.2020
114. Global Kids Online (2021). Digital Environment 2021. Available from: http://globalkidsonline.net/wp-content/uploads/2021/04/Digital-environment-REV.pdf. Accessed 28.04.2022
115. Gonçalves LS, Wolff L, Staggers N, Peres A (2012). Nursing informatics competencies: an analysis of the latest research. 2012;2012:127
116. Gopalan SS, Mohanty S, Das A (2012). Assessing community health workers' performance motivation: a mixed-methods approach on India's Accredited Social Health Activists (ASHA) programme. BMJ Open. 2:e001557
117. Government of the Republic of Korea (2020). Flattening the Curve on Covid 19: How Korea Responded to a Pandemic Using ICT. The Government of the Republic of Korea. Available from: http://www.undp.org/content/seoul_policy_center/en/home/presscenter/articles/2019/flattening-the-curve-on-covid-19.html. Accessed 14.03.2020
118. Gray K (2016). Public Health Platforms: An Emerging Informatics Approach to Health Professional Learning and Development. J Public Health Res 26;5(1):665. doi: 10.4081/jphr.2016.665
119. Gray K, Choo D, Butler-Henderson K, Whetton S, Maeder A (2015). Clinical Informatics Education. An online health informatics subject for clinical health profession students in Australian universities: an extension of the OLT Priority Project Coordinated interprofessional curriculum renewal for ehealth capability in clinical health profession degrees. Final report Available from: http://clinicalinformaticseducation.pbworks.com/w/file/fetch/103478171/ Clinical%20Informatics%20and%20eHealth%20OLT%20Final%20Report%202015.pdf. Accessed 12.02.2022
120. Gray K, Dattakumar A, Maeder A, Butler-Henderson K, Chenery H (2014). Advancing E-health education for the clinical health professions. Available from: http://clinicalinformaticseducation.pbworks.com/w/file/fetch/ 74500403/PP10_1806_Gray_report_2014.pd. Accessed 10.09.2022
121. Greenhalgh T, Wherton J, Shaw S, Morrison C (2020). Video consultations for covid-19. BMJ. 368:m998

122. Greenhalgh T, Robert G, Macfarlane F, Bate P, Kyriakidou O (2004). Diffusion of innovations in service organizations: systematic review and recommendations. Milbank Q. 2004;82(4):581–629. pmid:15595944

123. Griebel, L., et al. (2018). eHealth literacy research-Quo vadis? Inform Health Soc Care. 43(4): p. 427-442. Available from: https://doi.org/10.1080/17538157.2017.1364247. Accessed 05.04.2022

124. Griffin. (2021). Available from https://www.griffinbenefits.com/blog/five-telehealth-trends-for-2021. Accessed 20.04.2022

125. GSM Association. The State of Mobile Internet Connectivity 2020. Available from: https://www.gsma.com/r/wp-content/uploads/2020/09/GSMA-State-of-Mobile-Internet-Connectivity-Report-2020.pdf. Accessed 13.04.22

126. Haile F, Yemane D, Gebreslassie A (2014). Assessment of non-financial incentives for volunteer community health workers - the case of Wukro district, Tigray, Ethiopia. Hum Resour Health. 12:54–60

127. Hajat et al. (2018). Preventive Medicine Report 12, 284-293.

128. Han YY, Carcillo JA, Venkataraman ST, Clark RSB, Watson RS, Nguyen TC, et al. (2005). Unexpected increased mortality after implementation of a commercially sold computerized physician order entry system. Pediatrics 116(6):1506-12.

129. Han ER, Yeo S, Kim M-J, Lee Y-H, Park K-H, Roh H (2019). Medical education trend for future physicians in the era of advanced technology and artificial intelligence: an integrative review. BMC Med Educ 19(1):460.

130. Hancock VE. US Department of Education (1993). Information Literacy for Lifelong Learning Available from: https://files.eric.ed.gov/fulltext/ED358870.pdf. Accessed 10.02.2022

131. Harris, K., G. Jacobs, and J. Reeder (2019). Health Systems and Adult Basic Education: A Critical Partnership in Supporting Digital Health Literacy.Health Lit Res Pract. 3(3 Suppl): p. S33-s36. Available from: https://doi.org/10.3928/24748307-20190325-02. Accessed 05.04.2022

132. Health Data Collaborative (2018). Health Data Collaborative Secretariat, Health Data Collaborative Progress Report 2016–18. Available from: https://www.healthdatacollaborative.org/fileadmin/uploads/hdc/Documents/HDC_Progress_Report_Update_AW_071218_Web.pdf. Accessed 03.03.2022

133. Health Data Collaborative (2020). Where We Work. Health Data Collaborative. Available from: https://www.healthdatacollaborative.org/where-we-work/. Accessed 03.03.2022

134. Health Information Technology Competencies (2020). Available from: http://hitcomp.org/competencies/. Accessed 16.03.2022

135. Hermann K, Van Damme W, Pariyo GW, Schouten E, Assefa Y, Cirera A,

136. Hidalgo A, Gabaly S, Morales-Alonso G, Urueña A (2020). The digital divide in light of sustainable development: An approach through advanced machine learning techniques. Technol Forecast Soc Change [Internet]. 2020 [cited 2021 Nov 10];150(C). Available from: https://econpapers.repec.org/article/eeetefoso/v_3a150_3ay_3a2020_3ai_3ac_3as0040162519. Accessed 28.04.2022

137. Hillestad R, Bigelow J, Bower A, Girosi F, Meili R, Scoville R, et al. (2005). Can electronic medical record systems transform health care? Potential health benefits, savings, and costs. *Health Aff (Millwood)* 24:1103–7

138. Hilty DM, Crawford A, Teshima J, Chan S, Sunderji N, Yellowlees PM, et al. (2015). A framework for telepsychiatric training and e-health: competency-based education, evaluation and implications. Int Rev Psychiatry 27(6):569-592

139. HIMSS. Available from https://www.himss.org/resources/interoperability-healthcare. Accessed 20.04.2022

140. Holst C, Sukums F, Radovanovic D, Ngowi B, Noll J, Winkler A (2020). Sub-Saharan Africa-the new breeding ground for global digital health. Lancet Digital Health Apr;2(4):160-162

141. Honey ML, Skiba DJ, Procter P, Foster J, Kouri P, Nagle LM (2017). Nursing Informatics Competencies for Entry to Practice: The Perspective of Six Countries. Stud Health Technol Inform 232:51-61

142. Honeyman M, Maguire D, Evans H, Davies A (2020). Digital technology and health inequalities: a scoping review [Internet].Cardiff: Public Health Wales NHS Trust; p. 44. Available from: https://phw.nhs.wales/publications/publications1/digital-technology-and-health-inequalities-a-scoping-review/. Accessed 28.04.2022

143. Hsu W, Chiang C, Yang S (2014). The effect of individual factors on health behaviors among college students: the mediating effects of eHealth literacy. J Med Internet Res 16(12):e287

144. https://apps.who.int/iris/rest/bitstreams/1256930/retrieve. Accessed 08.05.2022

145. Hübner U, Shaw T, Thye J, Egbert N, Marin H, Ball M (2016). Towards an international framework for recommendations of core competencies in nursing and interprofessional informatics: the tiger competency synthesis project. Stud Health Technol Inform 228:655-659.

146. Hübner U, Shaw T, Thye J, Egbert N, Marin HD, Chang P, et al (2018). Technology informatics guiding education reform - tiger. Methods Inf Med 57(S 01):e30-e42

147. Hübner U, Thye J, Shaw T, Elias B, Egbert N, Saranto K, et al (2019). Towards the tiger international framework for recommendations of core competencies in health informatics 2.0: extending the scope and the roles. Stud Health Technol Inform 264:1218-1222

148. Hübner U, Thye J, Shaw T, Elias B, Egbert N, Saranto K, et al (2019). Towards the tiger international framework for recommendations of core competencies in health informatics 2.0: extending the scope and the roles. Stud Health Technol Inform 21;264:1218-1222

149. Hwang HG, Chen RF, Chang LH, Hsiao JL (2008). A study of the informatics literacy of clinical nurses in Taiwan. Comput Inform Nurs 26(5):290-299

150. Institute of Medicine (2003). *Key Capabilities of an Electronic Health Record System: Letter Report.* Washington, DC: The National Academies Press; pp. 1–36

151. International Organization for Standardization (2005). ISO/DTC 20514. *Health Informatics-Electronic Health Record-Defination, Scope, and Context 2005.* Available from: https://www.iso.org/obp/ui/#iso:std:39525:en. Accessed 23.04.2022

152. International Standardization Organization (ISO). 2019. Ergonomics of human-system interaction - Part 210: Human-centred design for interactive systems. Available from: https://www.iso.org/obp/ui/#iso:std:iso:9241:-210:ed-2:v1:en. Accessed 14.04.2022

153. International Telecommunication Union (2020). Measuring Digital Development: Facts and Figures 2020. Geneva, Switzerland: International Telecommunications Union. Available from: https://www.itu.int/en/ITU-D/Statistics/Pages/ff2020interactive.aspx. Accessed 28.04.2022

154. International Telecommunications Union (2015). ICT Facts & Figures: The World in 2015. Geneva: International Telecommunications Union.

155. International Telecommunications Union (2018). New ITU statistics show more than half the world is now using the Internet. ITU News. Available from: https://news.itu.int/itu-statistics-leaving-no-one-offline/. Accessed 02.03.2022

156. International Telecommunications Union (2019). Mobile cellular networks now cover most of the planet, with 97 percent of the global population within reach of a mobile signal, and at least 93 percent of the global population able to access 3G or higher mobile broadband services. Doreen Bogdan-Martin, "Measuring digital development: Facts & figures. ITU News. Available from: https://news.itu.int/measuring-digital-development-facts-figures-2019/. Accessed 02.03.2022

157. Ishikawa H, Takeuchi T, Yano E (2008). Measuring functional, communicative, and critical health literacy among diabetic patients. Diabetes Care. 31(5):874-879

158. Jerving S (2019). Data gaps threaten achievement of development goals in Africa. *DevEx News*. Available from: https://www.devex.com/news/data-gaps-threaten-achievement-of-development-goals-in-africa-95825; Accessed 03.03.2022

159. Jidkov L, Alexander M, Bark P, Williams JG, Kay J, Taylor P, et al. (2019) . Health informatics competencies in postgraduate medical education and training in the UK: a mixed methods study. BMJ Open 9(3):e025460

160. Jimoh L, Pate MA, Lin L, Schulman KA (2012). A model for the adoption of ICT by health workers in Africa. *Int J Med Inform.* 81:773–81

161. Jogerst K, Callender B, Adams V, Evert J, Fields E, Hall T, et al (2015). Identifying interprofessional global health competencies for 21st-century health professionals. Ann Glob Health 81(2):239-247

162. Joint Research Centre (European Commission), Brande LV den, Carretero S, Vuorikari R, Punie Y (2017). DigComp 2.0: the digital competence framework for citizens. LU: Publications Office of the European Union; 2017. Available from: https://data.europa.eu/doi/10.2791/11517. Accessed 28.04.2022

163. Jolly R. Parliament of Australia (2011). The e health revolution - easier said than done. Available from: https://www.aph.gov.au/ about_parliament/parliamentary_departments/parliamentary_library/pubs/rp/rp1112/12rp03. Accessed 10.02.2022

164. Journal of Clinical Nursing, 28 (5–6), 745–761

165. Kamadjeu RM, Tapang EM, Moluh RN (2005). Designing and implementing an electronic health record system in primary care practice in sub-Saharan Africa: A case study from Cameroon. *Inform Prim Care.* 13:179–86

166. Kapologwe N, Kibusi S, Borghi J, Gwajima D and kalolo A (2020). BMC Health Services Research. 20:104 Available from: https://doi.org/10.1186/s12913-020-4961-9. Accessed 06.02.2022

167. Kayser, L., et al. (2018). A Multidimensional Tool Based on the eHealth Literacy Framework: Development and Initial Validity Testing of the eHealth Literacy Questionnaire (eHLQ). J Med Internet Res. 20(2): p. e36. Available from: https://doi.org/10.2196/jmir.8371. Accessed 05.04.2022

168. Keasberry J, Scott IA, Sullivan C, Staib A, Ashby R (2017). Going digital: a narrative overview of the clinical and organisational impacts of eHealth technologies in hospital practice. Aust Health Rev Dec;41(6):646-664

169. Keesara S, Jonas A, Schulman K. Covid-19 and health care 's digital revolution. N Engl J Med. 2020;382:e82.

170. Khurana M (2020). Keeping pace: the need for digital health education in medical schools. Acad Med. 95(11):1629–30. Available from: https://journals.lww.com/10.1097/ACM.0000000000003672. Accessed 22.03.2022

171. Kickbusch I, Piselli D, Agrawal A, Balicer R, Banner O, Adelhardt M, et al (2021). The Lancet and Financial Times Commission on governing health futures 2030: growing up in a digital world. The Lancet. Oct;1–50

172. Kim H, Kim SY, Joly Y (2018). South Korea: in the midst of a privacy reform centered on data sharing. Available from: https://www.ncbi.nlm.nih.gov/pmc/articles/PMC6132641/. Accessed 05.03.2022

173. Klecun E, Lichtner V, Cornford T (2014). e-Literacy in health care. Stud Health Technol Inform 205:843-847.

174. Konttila, J., Siira, H., Kyngäs, H., Lahtinen, M., Elo, S., Kääriäinen, M., Kaakinen, O., Oikarinen, A., Yamakawa, M., Fukui, S., Utsumi, M., Higami, Y., Higuchi, A., & Mikkonen, K. (2018). Healthcare professionals' competence in digitalisation: A systematic review.

175. Koonin et al. (2020). Centers for Disease Control and Prevention 69, 1595-1599

176. Kreofsky. (2020). Available from https://pivotpointconsulting.com/insights/blog/the-future-of-telehealth-is-now-4-key-trends-for-2021/. Accessed 20.04.2022

177. Krumholz H (2014). Time To Assess Pharma Progress In Data Sharing. *Forbes*. Available from: https://www.forbes.com/sites/harlankrumholz/2014/06/02/time-to-assess-pharma-progress-in-data-sharing/. Accessed 03.03.2022

178. Kujala, S., Rajalahti, E., Heponiemi, T., & Hilama, P. (2018). Health professionals' expanding eHealth competences for supporting patients' self-management. Studies in Health Technology and Informatics, 247, 181–185

179. Kumar S, Preetha G (2012). Health promotion: an effective tool for global health. Indian J Community Med 37(1):5-12

180. Kumari et al. (2020). Somatosensory & Motor Research 38, 117-126

181. Lam M, Hines M, Lowe R, Nagarajan S, Keep M, Penman M, et al. (2016) Preparedness for eHealth: Health Sciences Students' Knowledge, Skills, and Confidence. JITE:Research 15:305-334. [doi: 10.28945/3523]

182. Laukka, E., Huhtakangas, M., Heponiemi, T., Kujala, S., Kaihlanen, A.-M., Gluschkoff, K., & Kanste, O. (2020). Health care professionals' experiences of patient-professional communication over patient portals: Systematic review of qualitative studies. Journal of Medical Internet Research, 22 (12), e21623

183. Lee, J.-A., et al. (2018). *Effective behavioral intervention strategies using mobile health applications for chronic disease management: a systematic review.* BMC medical informatics and decision making. 18(1): p. 12-12. Available from: https://doi.org/10.1186/s12911-018-0591-0. Accessed 05.04.2022

184. Lehne, M., Sass, J., Essenwanger, A. *et al. (2019).* Why digital medicine depends on interoperability. *npj Digit. Med.* 2, 79. https://doi.org/10.1038/s41746-019-0158-1

185. Lennon MR, Bouamrane M-M, Devlin AM, O'Connor S, O'Donnell C, Chetty U, et al. (2017). Readiness for delivering digital health at scale: Lessons from a longitudinal qualitative evaluation of a National Digital Health Innovation Program in the United Kingdom. J Med Internet Res.16;19(2):e42

186. Li S, Bamidis PD, Konstantinidis ST, Traver V, Car J, Zary N. Setting priorities for EU healthcare workforce IT skills competence improvement. Health Informatics J 2017 Apr 01:1460458217704257. [doi: 10.1177/1460458217704257]

187. Loftus P (2019). Drugmakers Turn to Data Mining to Avoid Expensive, Lengthy Drug Trials. The Wall Street Journal. Available from: https://www.wsj.com/articles/drugmakers-turn-to-data-mining-to-avoid-expensive-lengthy-drug-trials-11577097000; Accessed 28.02.2022

188. Luga et al. (2014). Risk Management and Healthcare Policy 7, 35-44

189. Lupton, D. (2017). Digital health now and in the future: Findings from a participatory design stakeholder workshop. Digital Health, 3, 2055207617740018.

190. Maheu MM, Drude KP, Hertlein KM, Lipschutz R, Wall K, Hilty DM (2018). Correction to: an interprofessional framework for telebehavioral health competencies. J Technol Behav Sci 5;3(2):108-140

191. Mahmood, A., et al. (2019). *Use of mobile health applications for health-promoting behavior among individuals with chronic medical conditions.* Digital Health. 5: p. Available from: 2055207619882181-2055207619882181. https://doi.org/10.1177/2055207619882181. Accessed 05.04.2022

192. Mai MV, Luo BT, Orenstein EW, Luberti AA. A model for clinical informatics education for residents: Addressing an unmet need. Appl Clin Inform. 2018;9(2):261-7

193. Mandl KD, Kohane IS. Tectonic shifts in the health information economy. N Engl J Med. 2008;358(16):1732-7

194. Mantas J, Ammenwerth E, Demiris G, Hasman A, Haux R, Hersh W (2010). IMIA Recommendations on Education Task Force. Recommendations of the international medical informatics association (IMIA) on education in biomedical and health informatics. First revision. Methods Inf Med 49(2):105-120

195. Marcos Y, Phelps BR, Bachman G. Community strategies that improve care and retention along the prevention of mother-to-child transmission of HIV cascade: a review. J Int AIDS Soc. 2012;15:17394.

196. Marotta C. Motivational aspects and level of satisfaction of Italian junior doctors with regard to knowledge and skills acquired attending specific general practice training courses. A national web survey. EuroMediterr Biomed J. 2017;(12):77-86

197. Mattson, T. (2016). eHealth and the law. In G. Erlingsdóttir, & H. Sandberg (Eds.), eHealth opportunities and challenges: A white paper (pp. 13–18). The Pufendorf Institute of Advanced Studies, Lund University

198. McCoy LG, Nagaraj S, Morgado F, Harish V, Das S, Celi LA (2020). What do medical students actually need to know about artificial intelligence? NPJ Digit Med. 2020;3(1):86. Available from: http://www.nature.com/articles/s41746-020-0294-7.

199. Mechael P, Edelman JK (2019). The State of Digital Health 2019. Washington, D.C.: Health Enabled and Global Development Incubator. Available from: https://www.digitalhealthindex.org/stateofdigitalhealth19. Accessed 02.03.2022

200. Meldolesi E, van Soest J, Alitto AR, Autorino R, Dinapoli N, Dekker A, et al (2014).. VATE: VAlidation of high TEchnology based on large database analysis by learning machine. Colorectal Cancer. 1;3(5):435-50

201. Merritt K, Smith KD, Di Renzo JC (2005). An investigation of self-reported computer literacy: is it reliable? *Issues Inf Syst.* 6(1):289–95.

202. Mesko B, Győrffy Z, Kollár J (2015). Digital literacy in the medical curriculum: a course with social media tools and gamification. JMIR Med Educ 1;1(2):e6

203. Mian A, Khan S (2020). Medical education during pandemics: a UK perspective. BMC Med 9;18(1):100

204. Mikkonen, K., Ojala, T., Sjögren, T., Piirainen, A., Koskinen, C., Koskinen, M., Koivula, M., Sormunen, M., Saaranen, T., Salminen, L., Koskimäki, M., Ruotsalainen, H., Lähteenmäki, M.-L., Wallin, O., Mäki-Hakola, H., & Kääriäinen, M. (2018). Competence areas of health science teachers -a systematic review of quantitative studies. Nurse Education Today, 70 , 77–86

205. Ministry of Health and Social Welfare (2015). The United Republic of Tanzania. Health Sector Strategic Plan July 2015 – June 2020 (HSSP IV). Available from: https://tinyurl.com/46mz24h4. Accessed 13.04.2022

206. Ministry of Health and Social Welfare (2015). The United Republic of Tanzania. The National Strategic Plan V (2015-2020) for Tuberculosis and Leprosy. Available from: https://ntlp.go.tz/site/assets/files/1074/national_strategic_plan_2015_2020.pdf. Accessed 14.04.2022

207. Ministry of Health, Community Development, Gender, Elderly and Children (2017). he United Republic of Tanzania. National Aids Control Programme. National Guidelines for the Management of HIV and AIDS. Available from: https://tinyurl.com/r9emcp34. Accessed 14.04.2022

208. Ministry of Health, Community Development, Gender, Elderly and Children (2019).The United Republic of Tanzania. Digital Health Strategy, July 2019 - June 2024. Available from: http://moh.go.tz/en/strategic-plans?download=395:digital-health-strategy. Accessed 14.04.2022

209. Mobile Ecosystem Forum (2015). Global mHealth & Wearables Report 2015. Available from: https://mobileecosystemforum.com/mef-global-mhealth-and-wearables-report-2015/. Accessed 28.02.2022

210. Mohsin-Shaikh S, Furniss D, Blandford A, McLeod M, Ma T, Beykloo MY, et al (2019). The impact of electronic prescribing systems on healthcare professionals' working practices in the hospital setting: a systematic review and narrative synthesis. BMC Health Serv Res Oct 22;19(1):742

211. Mohsin-Shaikh S, Furniss D, Blandford A, McLeod M, Ma T, Beykloo MY, et al. The impact of electronic prescribing systems on healthcare professionals' working practices in the hospital setting: a systematic review and narrative synthesis. BMC Health Serv Res 2019 Oct 22;19(1):742

212. Monda J, Keipeer J, Were MC (2012). Data integrity module for data quality assurance within an e-health system in sub-Saharan Africa. *Telemed J E Health.* 18:5–10

213. Morris D (2015). Russia's Personal Data Localization Law Goes Into Effect. Available from: http://www.duanemorris.com/alerts/russia_personal_data_localization_law_goes_into_effect_1015.html?utm_

source=Mondaq&utm_medium=syndication&utm_campaign=View-Original. Accessed 05.03.2022

214. Murphy PW, Davis TC, Long SW, Jackson RH, Decker BC. Rapid Estimate of Adult Literacy in Medicine (REALM): a quick reading test for patients. J Read 1993 Oct;37(2):124-130

215. Mwakapeje ER, Høgset S, Fyumagwa R, Nonga HE, Mdegela RH, Skjerve E (2018). Anthrax outbreaks in the humans - livestock and wildlife interface areas of Northern Tanzania: a retrospective record review 2006-2016. BMC Public Health 2018 Jan 05;18(1):106

216. Nagle LM, Crosby K, Frisch N, Borycki E, Donelle L, Hannah K, et al (2014). Developing entry-to-practice nursing informatics competencies for registered nurses. Stud Health Technol Inform ;201:356-363

217. Nanah A, Bayoumi AB (2020). The pros and cons of digital health communication tools in neurosurgery: a systematic review of literature. Neurosurg Rev 43(3):835-846

218. National Bureau of Statistics (2018).The United Republic of Tanzania. Tanzania in figures. Available from: https://www.nbs.go.tz/nbs/takwimu/references/Tanzania_in_Figures_2018.pdf. Accessed 14.04.2022

219. National E-Health Transition Authority (2016). Evolution of eHealth in Australia: Achievements, Lessons, and Opportunities. Sydney. Available from: https://tinyurl.com/yy3xg947. Accessed 14.03.2022

220. National House Ordinance of the People's Republic of China No. 717, (2019). Available from: http://www.gov.cn/zhengce/content/2019-06/10/content_5398829.htm; Accessed 05.03.2022

221. National Institute of Mental Health. (2021). Available from https://www.nimh.nih.gov/health/statistics/mental-illness. Accessed 20.04.2022

222. Nazeha N, Pavagadhi, D., Kyaw, B. M., Car, J., Jimenez, G., and Car, L. T. (2020). A digitally competent health workforce: Scoping review of educational frameworks. Journal of Medical Internet Research, 22 (11), e22706

223. NEJM Catalyst. (2018). Available from: https://catalyst.nejm.org/doi/full/10.1056/CAT.18.0268. Accessed 20.04.2022

224. Neter E and Brainin E (2012). eHealth literacy: extending the digital divide to the realm of health information. J Med Internet Res 14(1):e19

225. Neter E, Brainin E, Baron-Epel O (2015). The dimensionality of health literacy and eHealth literacy. *Eur Health Psychol.* 17(6):275–80.

226. New J (2019). The Promise of Data-Driven Drug Development. Center for Data Innovation. Available from: https://www.datainnovation.org/2019/09/the-promise-of-data-driven-drug-development/. Accessed 28.02.2022

227. Ngowi HA, Winkler AS, Braae UC, Mdegela RH, Mkupasi EM, Kabululu ML, et al. (2019). Taenia solium taeniosis and cysticercosis literature in Tanzania provides research evidence justification for control: A systematic scoping review. PLoS One 14(6):e0217420

228. Norgaard O, Furstrand D, Klokker L, Karnoe A, Batterham R, Kayser L, et al (2015). The e-health literacy framework: a conceptual framework for characterizing e-health users and their interaction with e-health systems. Knowl Manag E-Learn 7(4):522-540

229. Norman C (2011). eHealth literacy 2.0: problems and opportunities with an evolving concept. *J Med Internet Res.* 13(4):e125. doi: 10.2196/jmir.2035

230. Norman CD and Skinner HA (2006). eHealth Literacy: essential Skills for Consumer Health in a Networked World. J Med Internet Res 8(2):e9

231. Novoa, R. B. (2021). State of the Art and Future Applications of Digital Health in Chile. *International journal of health & medical sciences*

232. Nutbeam D. World Health Organization (1998). Health Promotion Glossary. Available from: http://www.who.int/healthpromotion/about/HPR%20Glossary%201998.pdf?ua=1. Accessed 06.04.2022

233. O'Leary KJ, Liebovitz DM, Feinglass J, Liss DT, Evans DB, Kulkarni N, et al. Creating a better discharge summary: Improvement in quality and timeliness using an electronic discharge summary. J Hosp Med. 2009;4(4):219–25

234. Obermeyer Z, Emanuel EJ. Predicting the future – Big data, machine learning, and clinical medicine. N Engl J Med. 2016;375(13):1216-9

235. Obermeyer Z, Lee TH. Lost in Thought - The Limits of the Human Mind and the Future of Medicine. N Engl J Med 2017 Sep 28;377(13):1209-1211. Available from: [doi: 10.1056/NEJMp1705348]. Accessed 10.02.2022

236. O'Connell J, Gardner G, Coyer F. Beyond competencies: using a capability framework in developing practice standards for advanced practice nursing. J Adv Nurs 2014 Dec;70(12):2728-2735

237. Odendaal WA, Anstey Watkins J, Leon N, Goudge J, Griffiths F, Tomlinson M, Daniels K. Health workers' perceptions and experiences of using mHealth technologies to deliver primary healthcare services: a qualitative evidence synthesis. Cochrane Database Syst Rev. 2020 Mar 26;3(3):CD011942. doi: 10.1002/14651858.CD011942.pub2. PMID: 32216074; PMCID: PMC7098082.

238. Odone A, Buttigieg S, Ricciardi W, Azzopardi-Muscat N, Staines A (2019). Public health digitalization in Europe. Eur J Public Health. 1;29(Supplement_3):28–35. pmid:31738441

239. OECD (2020), Beyond Containment: Health systems responses to COVID19 in the OECD, OECD Publishing, Paris. Available from: https://oe.cd/covid19briefhealth. Accessed 28.04.2022

240. Office for National Statistics (United Kingdom) (2019). Exploring the UK's digital divide. Report No.: March. Available from: http://globalkidsonline.net/wp-content/uploads/2021/04/Digital-environment-REV.pdf. Accessed 28.04.2022

241. Oluoch T, Santas X, Kwaro D, Were M, Biondich P, Bailey C, et al (2012). The effect of electronic medical record-based clinical decision support on HIV care in resource-constrained settings: A systematic review. *Int J Med Inform.* 81:e83–92

242. Osborne RH, Batterham RW, Elsworth GR, Hawkins M, Buchbinder R (2013). The grounded psychometric development and initial validation of the Health Literacy Questionnaire (HLQ). BMC Public Health 13:658

243. Pantuvo JS, Naguib R, Wickramasinghe N (2011). Towards implementing a nationwide electronic health record system in Nigeria. *Int J Healthc Deliv Reform Initiatives.* 3:39–55.

244. Parker RM, Baker DW, Williams MV, Nurss JR 81995). The test of functional health literacy in adults: a new instrument for measuring patients' literacy skills. J Gen Intern Med 10(10):537-541

245. Pathipati AS, Azad TD, Jethwani K (2016). Telemedical education: training digital natives in telemedicine. J Med Internet Res 12;18(7):e193

246. Peckham D (2016). Electronic patient records, past, present and future. Paediatr Respir Rev Aug(20 Suppl):8-11

247. Pennic (2020). Available from https://hitconsultant.net/2021/01/04/telehealth-virtual-care-predictions-trends-2021/#.YRpgiogzaUk. Accessed 20.04.2022

248. Perez F, Ba H, Dastagire SG, Altmann M. The role of community health workers in improving child health programmes in Mali. BMC Int Health Hum Rights. 2009;9:28–40

249. Personally Controlled Electronic Health Records (2012). Australia. Available from: https://www.legislation.gov.au/Details/C2012A00063. Accessed 05.02.2022

250. Petersen T, Steiner F (2019). Megatrend-Report #01: The Bigger Picture [Internet]. Gütersloh: Bertelsmann Stiftung. Available from: https://www.bertelsmann-stiftung.de/en/publications/publication/did/the-bigger-picture-1. Accessed 28.04.2022

251. Pew Research Center (2018). Internet connectivity seen as having positive impact on life in Sub-Saharan Africa. Available from: https://www.pewresearch.org/global/2018/10/09/majorities-in-sub-saharan-africa-own-mobile-phones-but-smartphone-adoption-is-modest/. Accessed 14.08.2022

252. Phaneuf (2021). Available from https://www.businessinsider.com/wearable-technology-healthcare-medical-devices?r=US&IR=T. Accessed 20.04.2022

253. Phelps R, Hase S, Ellis A. Competency, capability, complexity and computers: exploring a new model for conceptualizing end-user computer education. Br J Educ Technol 2005 Jan;36(1):67-84

254. Poncette A-S, Glauert DL, Mosch L, Braune K, Balzer F, Back DA (2020). Undergraduate medical competencies in digital health and curricular module development: mixed methods study. J Med Internet Res. 2020;22(10):e22161. Available from: http://www.jmir.org/2020/10/e22161/. Accessed 22.03.2022

255. Praia Group (2014). Praia Group on Governance Statistics. Available from: http://www.ine.cv/praiagroup/. Accessed 03.03.2022

256. Price Waterhouse Coopers (2012). Emerging mHealth: Paths for Growth. Available from: https://www.pwc.com/gx/en/healthcare/mhealth/assets/pwc-emerging-mhealth-full.pdf. Accessed 28.02.2022

257. Price-Haywood, E.G., et al. (2017). eHealth Literacy: Patient Engagement in Identifying Strategies to Encourage Use of Patient Portals Among Older Adults. Popul Health Manag. 20(6): p. 486-494. Available from: https://doi.org/10.1089/pop.2016.0164. Accessed 05.04.2022

258. Procter PM. Ubiquitous Adoption of Innovative and Supportive Information and Communications Technology Across Health and Social Care Needs Education for Clinicians. Stud Health Technol Inform 2017;235:358-362

259. Purc-Stephenson, R., & Thrasher, C. (2010). Nurses' experiences with telephone triage and advice: A meta ethnography. Journal of Advanced Nursing, 66 (3), 482–494

260. Radovanović D, Holst C, Belur S, Srivastava R, Houngbonon G, Le Quentrec E, et al. (2020). Digital literacy key performance indicators for sustainable development. Soc Inclusion 14;8(2):151-167

261. Reserve Bank of India (2018). Frequently Asked Questions. RBI website, Available from: https://m.rbi.org.in/Scripts/FAQView.aspx?Id=130. Accessed 05.03.2022

262. Rice N, Robone S and Smith PC (2012). Vignettes and health systems responsiveness in cross-country comparative analyses. doi.org/10.1111/j.1467-985X.2011.01021. Available from: https://rss.onlinelibrary.wiley.com/doi/full/10.1111/j.1467-985X.2011.01021.x. Accessed 30.01.2022

263. Risling T (2019). Beyond the Divide: Exploring the Digital Determinants of Health. In: Canada Health Infoway: Infoway Partnership Conference. Available from: https://www.infoway-inforoute.ca/en/component/edocman/supporting-documents/partnership/3770-ipc2019-day02-1040-1110-tracie-risling-en-pdf?Itemid=101. Accessed 28.04.2022

264. Ritchie et al. (2018). Available from https://ourworldindata.org/mental-health#citation. Accessed 20.04.2022

265. Robbins, D. and P. Dunn (2019). Digital health literacy in a person-centric world. Int J Cardiol. 290: p. 154-155. Available from: https://doi.org/10.1016/j.ijcard.2019.05.033. Accessed 05.04.2022

266. Robinson SA, Larsen DE. The relative influence of the community and health system on work performance: a case study of community health workers in Colombia. Soc Sci Med. 1990;30:1041–8.

267. Rogers C (1951),. Client-centered therapy; its current practice, implications, and theory; Houghton Mifflin: Oxford, London, pp. xii, 560-xii, 560.

268. Röhrig R, Stausberg J, Dugas M, GMDS project group, Medical Informatics Education in Medicine. Development of national competency-based learning objectives "Medical Informatics" for

undergraduate medical education. Methods Inf Med 2013;52(3):184-188.

269. Rome Call For Ethics [Internet]. 2020. Available from: www.academyforlife.va/content/dam/pav/documenti%20pdf/2020/CALL%2028%20febbraio/AI%20Rome%20Call%20x%20firma_DEF_DEF_.pdf

270. Rosenman D, Swanson WS (2020). "Digital health" in medical school. Acad Med. 95(7):973–3. Available from: https://journals.lww.com/10.1097/ACM.0000000000003359. Accessed 22.03.2022

271. Ross, J., Stevenson, F., Lau, R., & Murray, E. (2016). Factors that influence the implementation of e-health: A systematic review of systematic reviews (an update). Implementation Science, 11, 146

272. Rotich JK, Hannan TJ, Smith FE, Bii J, Odero WW, Vu N, et al (2003). Installing and implementing a computer-based patient record system in sub-Saharan Africa: The Mosoriot Medical Record System. *J Am Med Inform Assoc.* 10:295–303

273. Royal College of Nursing (2017). Improving Digital Literacy. Available from: https://www.rcn.org.uk/professional-development/publications/pub-006129. Accessed 14.03.2022

274. Royal College of Nursing (2017). Improving Digital Literacy. Available from: https://www.rcn.org.uk/professional-development/publications/pub-006129. Accessed 31.03.2022

275. Rutledge et al. (2017). Advances in Medical Education and Practices 8, 399-409

276. Sarna A, Luchters S, Musenge E, Okal J, Chersich M, Tun W, et al. Effectiveness of a community-based positive prevention intervention for people living with HIV who are not receiving antiretroviral treatment: a prospective cohort study. Global Health Sci Practice. 2013;1:52–67

277. Schank RC, Berman TR. The pervasive role of stories in knowledge and action. In: Green MC, Strange JJ, Brock TC, editors. Narrative Impact: Social and Cognitive Foundations. New York: Lawrence Erlbaum Associates Publishers; 2002:287-313

278. Scheerder A, van Deursen A, van Dijk J (2017). Determinants of Internet skills, uses and outcomes. A systematic review of the second- and third-level digital divide. Telemat Inform. 34(8):1607–24

279. Schreiweis B, Pobiruchin M, Strotbaum V, Suleder J, Wiesner M, Bergh B (2019). Barriers and facilitators to the implementation of ehealth services: systematic literature analysis. J Med Internet Res 22;21(11):e14197

280. Shapiro M (2012). Patient-Generated Health Data (white paper prepared for Office of Policy and Planning, Office of the National Coordinator for Health Information Technology, RTI International. Available from: http://www.healthit.gov/sites/default/files/rti_pghd_whitepaper_april_2012.pdf. Accessed 03.03.2022

281. Shaw T, McGregor D, Brunner M, Keep M, Janssen A, Barnet S (2017). What is eHealth? Development of a Conceptual Model for eHealth: Qualitative Study with Key Informants. J Med Internet Res doi: 10.2196/jmir.8106

282. Shortliffe EH, Cimino JJ (2014). *Biomedical Informatics: Computer Applications in Healthcare and Biomedicine.* New York, NY: Springer; pp. 1–43

283. Sieck CJ, Sheon A, Ancker JS, Castek J, Callahan B, Siefer A (2021). Digital inclusion as a social determinant of health. Npj Digit Med. 17;4(1):1–3. pmid:33398041

284. Simba DO, Mwangu M (2004). Application of ICT in strengthening health information systems in developing countries in the wake of globalization. *Afr Health Sci.* 2004;4:194–8.

285. Smith R (2010). Strategies for coping with information overload. BMJ. 341(dec15 2):c7126–6. Available from: https://www.bmj.com/lookup/doi/10.1136/bmj.c7126. Accessed 22.03.2022

286. Soellner R, Huber S, Reder M (2014). The concept of eHealth literacy and its measurement: German translation of the eHEALS. *J Media Psychol.* Jan;26(1):29–38. doi: 10.1027/1864-1105/a000104.

287. Sonnier P. The fourth wave: Digital health - a new era of human progress. San Diego, California; 2017.

288. Sørensen K, Van den Broucke S, Fullam J, Doyle G, Pelikan J, Slonska Z (2012). (HLS-EU) Consortium Health Literacy Project European. Health literacy and public health: a systematic review and integration of definitions and models. BMC Public Health 12:80

289. Staggers N, Gassert CA, Curran C (2001). Informatics competencies for nurses at four levels of practice. J Nurs Educ 40(7):303-316.

290. Staggers N, Gassert CA, Curran C (2002). A Delphi study to determine informatics competencies for nurses at four levels of practice. Nurs Res 51(6):383-390.

291. Stanford Medicine (2020). 2020 Health Trends Report: The Rise of the Data-Driven Physician. Stanford Medicine. Available from: http://med.stanford.edu/content/dam/sm/school/documents/Health-Trends-Report/Stanford%20Medicine%20Health%20Trends%20Report%202020.pdf. Accessed 13.04.2022

292. Strudwick G, Nagle L, Kassam I, Pahwa M, Sequeira L (2019). Informatics competencies for nurse leaders: a scoping review. J Nurs Adm 49(6):323-330

293. Su Z, McDonnell D, Wen J, Kozak M, Abbas J, Šegalo S, et al (2021). Mental health consequences of COVID-19 media coverage: the need for effective crisis communication practices. Glob Health. Jan5;17(1):4. pmid:33402169

294. Susskind R, Susskind D. Harvard Business Review. 2016. Technology Will Replace Many Doctors, Lawyers, and Other Professionals. Available from: https://hbr.org/2016/10/robots-will-replace-doctors-lawyers-and-other-professionals. Accessed 12.02.2022

295. Tagliaferri L, Budrukkar A, Lenkowicz J, Cambeiro M, Bussu F, Guinot JL, et al. ENT COBRA ONTOLOGY: the covariates classification system proposed by the Head & Neck and Skin GEC-ESTRO Working Group for interdisciplinary standardized data collection in head and neck patient cohorts treated with interventional radiotherapy (brachytherapy). J Contemp Brachyther. 2018;10(3):260-6.

296. Tagliaferri L, Kovács G, Autorino R, Budrukkar A, Guinot JL, Hildebrand G, et al (2016). ENT COBRA (Consortium for Brachytherapy Data Analysis): interdisciplinary standardized data collection system for head and neck patients treated with interventional radiotherapy (brachytherapy). J Contemp Brachyther. 4:336-43.

297. Technology Informatics Guiding Education Reform. EU US eHealth Works to Improve Global Workforce Development. 2017. Available from: https://tutcris.tut.fi/portal/files/12978862/Eu_us_ehealth_workforce_development.pdf. Accessed 16.03.2022

298. The Lancet Digital Health (2021). Digital technologies: a new determinant of health. Lancet Digit Health. 2021 Nov 1;3(11):e684. pmid:34711372

299. Thilen. (2020) Available from https://www.modjoul.com/blog/a-brief-history-of-wearable-technology. Accessed 20.04.2022

300. Thye J, Shaw T, Hüsers J, Esdar M, Ball M, Babitsch B, et al (2018). What are inter-professional ehealth competencies? Stud Health Technol Inform 253:201-205.

301. Tippawan L, Porntip P, Sunittha S and Nurleesa O (2012). Health System Responsiveness for delivery care in Southern Thailand. International Journal for Quality in Health Care, 24, 2: 169–175. Available from: https://doi.org/10.1093/intqhc/mzr085. Accessed 30.01.2022

302. TNS Political and Social. Flash Eurobarometer 404 European Citizens' Digital Health Literacy. Brussels, Belgium: European Union; 2014.

303. Tolib M and Sumit K (2017). What is health systems responsiveness? Review of existing knowledge and proposed conceptual framework. Available from: https:// doi.org/10.1136/bmjgh-2017-000486. Accessed 30.01.2022

304. Topol EJ (2019). High-performance medicine: the convergence of human and artificial intelligence. Nat Med. 25(1):44-56

305. Topol Review (2019). Preparing the Healthcare Workforce to Deliver the Digital Future. The NHS Constitution. Available from: https://topol.hee.nhs.uk/. Accessed 14.03.2022

306. Tuckett DA, Boulton M, Olson C (1985). A New Approach to the Measurement of Patients' Understanding of What They Are Told in Medical Consultations. Journal of Health and Social Behavior. 10.2307/2136724.

307. Tudor Car L, Kyaw BM, Nannan Panday RS, van der Kleij R, Chavannes N, Majeed A, et al. (2021). Digital health training programs for medical students: scoping review. JMIR Med Educ. 7(3):e28275. Available from: https://mededu.jmir.org/2021/3/e28275. Accessed 22.02.2022

308. Tyson JE (2018). Private infrastructure financing in developing countries. Five challenges, five solutions. (working paper 536, Overseas Development Institute, London, August 2018). Available from: https://www.odi.org/sites/odi.org.uk/files/resource-documents/12366.pdf. Accessed 02.03.2022

309. United Nations Development Programme (2019). The 2019 Global Multidimensional Poverty Index (MPI). Available from:: http://hdr.undp.org/en/2019-MPI. Accessed 10.05.2022

310. Unwin T, de Bastion G (2009). Bridging the digital divide. In: Kitchin R, Thrift N, editors. International Encyclopedia of Human Geography. Elsevier; 191–7

311. Utidjian et al. (2016). Pediatric Clinic of North America 63, 367-378

312. Valentine N, Silva A, Kawabata K, Darby CH, Murray JLC, and Evans D (2003). Health system responsiveness: concepts, domains and organization. In: Murray CJL, Evans DB, editors. Health System Performance Assessment (Debates, Methods and Empiricism). 1st ed. Geneva: World Health Organization. PP 565–72

313. Van Belle JP (2018). Africa Data Revolution Report 2018: Status and Emerging Impact of Open Data in Africa. Geneva: World Wide Web Foundation. Available from: , https://webfoundation.org/docs/2019/03/Africa-data-revolution-report.pdf; Accessed 03.03.2022

314. Van De Belt T, Engelen LG, Berben SA, Schoonhoven L (2010). Definition of Health 2.0 and Medicine 2.0: a systematic review. *J Med Internet Res.* 12(2):e18. doi: 10.2196/jmir.1350.

315. van der Vaart R, Drossaert CH, de Heus HM, Taal E, van de Laar MA (2013). Measuring actual eHealth literacy among patients with rheumatic diseases: a qualitative analysis of problems encountered using Health 1.0 and Health 2.0 applications. *J Med Internet Res.* 15(2):e27. doi: 10.2196/jmir.2428

316. van der Vaart R, van Deursen AJ, Drossaert CH, Taal E, van Dijk JA, van de Laar MA (2011). Does the eHealth Literacy Scale (eHEALS) measure what it intends to measure? Validation of a Dutch version of the eHEALS in two adult populations. *J Med Internet Res.* 2011;13(4):e86. doi: 10.2196/jmir.1840

317. van der Vaart, R. and C. Drossaert (2017). Development of the Digital Health Literacy Instrument: Measuring a Broad Spectrum of Health 1.0 and Health 2.0 Skills. J Med Internet Res. 19(1): p. e27. Available from: https://doi.org/10.2196/jmir.6709. Accessed 05.04.2022

318. van Deursen AJ, van Dijk JA (2011). Internet skills performance tests: are people ready for eHealth? *J Med Internet Res.* 13(2):e35. doi: 10.2196/jmir.1581

319. van Dijk JAGM (2012). The Evolution of the Digital Divide - The Digital Divide Turns to Inequality of Skills and Usage.In: Bus J, Crompton M, Hildebrandt M, Metakides G, editors. Digital Enlightenment Yearbook 2012. Netherlands: IOS Press; p. 57–78

320. van Houwelingen CT, Moerman AH, Ettema RG, Kort HS, Ten Cate O (2016). Competencies required for nursing digital health activities: A Delphi-study. Nurse Educ Today. 39:50-62

321. van Kessel R., Hrzic R., O'Nuallain E., Weir E., Wong B.L.H., Anderson M., Baron-Cohen S., & Mossialos E (2022). The digital health paradox: international policy perspectives to address the increased health inequalities for people living with disabilities. J Med Internet Res

322. van Kessel, R., Wong, B. L. H., Rubinić, I., O'Nuallain, E., & Czabanowska, K. (2022). Is Europe prepared to go digital? Making the case for developing digital capacity: an exploratory analysis of Eurostat survey data. *PLOS Digital Health*, *1*(2), e0000013

323. Värri A, Blake R, Roberts J, Fenton S, Cleary M, Zacks S, et al. Transatlantic collection of health informatics competencies. FinJeHeW 2016 May 23;8(2-3):127-136

324. Vincens N, Emmelin M, Stafström M (2018). Social capital, income inequality and the social gradient in self-rated health in Latin America: A fixed effects analysis. Soc Sci Med 196:115-122

325. Viswananthan K, Hansen PM, Rahman MH, Steinhardt L, Edward A, Arwal SH, et al. Can community health workers increase coverage of reproductive health services? J Epidemiol Commun Health. 2011;66:894–900

326. Vuorikari, R., Punie, Y., Carretero Gomez, S., & Van den Brande, G. (2016). DigComp 2.0: The digital competence framework for citizens. Update Phase 1: The Conceptual Reference Model. Luxembourg: Publication Office of the European Union. EUR 27948 EN. Retrieved from: https://ec.europa.eu/jrc/en/publication/eur-scientific-and-technical-research-reports/digco20-digital-competence-framework-citizens-update-phase-1-conceptual-reference-model Cited 2020/09/01

327. Wagner E, Austin B, Von Korff, M (1996). Improving outcomes in chronic illness. Managed Care Quarterly, 4; 2, 12-15

328. Wartman SA, Combs CD (2019. Reimagining medical education in the age of AI. AMA J Ethics. 21(2):E146–52. Available from: https://journalofethics.ama-assn.org/article/reimagining-medical-education-age-ai/2019-02. Accessed 22.03.2022

329. Westra BL, Delaney CW, Delaney C (2008). Informatics competencies for nursing and healthcare leaders. AMIA Annu Symp Proc 6:804-808

330. While, A., & Dewsbury, G. (2011). Nursing and information communication technology (ICT): A discussion of trends and future directions. International Journal of Nursing Studies, 48 (10), 1302–1310

331. Willett et al. (2006). Disease Control Priorities in Developing Edition 2, Chapter 44

332. Williams F, Boren SA (2008). The role of the electronic medical record (EMR) in care delivery development in developing countries: A systematic review. *Inform Prim Care.* 16:139–45

333. Williams F, Boren SA (2008). The role of the electronic medical record (EMR) in care delivery development in developing countries: A systematic review. *Inform Prim Care* 16:139–45

334. Wong BLH, Gray W, Holly L (2021). The future of health governance needs youth voices at the forefront. The Lancet. 1–2. pmid:34706261

335. World Bank (2021). Tanzania. Available from: https://www.worldbank.org/en/country/tanzania/overview#1. Accessed 13.04.2022

336. World Health Organization (2000). Measuring health system Responsiveness. World Health Report 2000. Geneva. Available from: http://www.who.int/responsiveness/papers/paper23.pdf. Accessed 30.01.2022

337. World Health Organization (2008). *Core Health Indicators*. Available from: http://www.apps.who.int/whosis/database/core/core_select_process.cfm. Accessed 23.04.2022

338. World Health Organization (2015). Atlas of eHealth country profiles: The use of eHealth in support of universal health coverage. Available from: https://www.who.int/publications-detail/atlas-of-ehealth-country-profiles-the-use-of-ehealth-in-support-of-universal-health-coverage. Accessed 01.03.2022

339. World Health Organization (2016): Global Diffusion of Ehealth: Making Universal Health Coverage Achievable. World Health Organization. Available from: https://apps.who.int/iris/bitstream/handle/10665/252529/9789241511780-eng.pdf?sequence=1. Accessed 14.03.2022

340. World Health Organization (2018). Digital Technologies: Shaping the Future of Primary Health Care, WHO, Geneva, Switzerland, 2018

341. World Health Organization (2019). Bangladesh's digital health journey: reflections on a decade of quiet revolution. Available from:

342. World Health Organization (2019). WHO Guideline: Recommendations on Digital Interventions for Health System Strengthening, World Health Organization, Geneva, Switzerland, 2019. Contract No.: License: CC BY-NC-SA 3.0 IGO

343. World Health Organization (2020). Global Strategy on Digital Health 2020-2025. Available from:https://www.who.int/docs/default-source/documents/gs4dhdaa2a9f352b0445bafbc79ca799dce4d.pdf. Accessed 25.02.2022

344. World Health Organization (2021). Taeniasis/cysticercosis. Available from: https://www.who.int/news-room/fact-sheets/detail/taeniasis-cysticercosis. Accessed 14.04.2022

345. World Wide Web Foundation (2018). Closing the Investment Gap: How Multilateral Development Banks Can Contribute to Digital Inclusion. Available from: https://webfoundation.org/research/closing-the-investment-gap-how-multilateral-development-banks-can-contribute-to-digital-inclusion/. Accessed 02.03.2022

346. Xie B (2011). Effects of an eHealth literacy intervention for older adults. J Med Internet Res 13(4):e90

347. Yan, K., C. Balijepalli, and E. Druyts (2021). The Impact of Digital Therapeutics on Current Health Technology Assessment Frameworks. Front Digit Health. 3: p. 667016. Available from: https://doi.org/10.3389/fdgth.2021.667016. Accessed 05.04.2022

348. Yarnell (2020). Available from https://www.bluestreamhealth.com/top-5-telehealth-trends-for-2021/. Accessed 20.04.2022

349. Zelezny-Green R, Vosloo S, Conole G. Digital inclusion for low-skilled and low-literate people: a landscape review. United Nations Educational, Scientific and Cultural Organization. 2018. Available from: https://unesdoc.unesco.org/ark:/48223/pf0000261791. Accessed 13.04.2022

INDEX

L

M

N

P

R

S

T

V

W

X